Leveraging Longitudinal Data in Developing Countries
Report of a Workshop

Workshop on Leveraging Longitudinal Data in Developing Countries Committee

Committee on Population

Valerie L. Durrant and Jane Menken, *Editors*

Division of Behavioral and Social Sciences and Education

National Research Council

NATIONAL ACADEMY PRESS
Washington, DC

NATIONAL ACADEMY PRESS   2101 Constitution Avenue, N.W.   Washington, DC 20418

NOTICE: The project that is the subject of this report was approved by the Governing Board of the National Research Council, whose members are drawn from the councils of the National Academy of Sciences, the National Academy of Engineering, and the Institute of Medicine. The members of the committee responsible for the report were chosen for their special competences and with regard for appropriate balance.

The study was supported by Contract/Grant No. 29900629 between the National Academy of Sciences and the Andrew W. Mellon Foundation. Any opinions, findings, conclusions, or recommendations expressed in this publication are those of the author(s) and do not necessarily reflect the view of the organizations or agencies that provided support for this project.

International Standard Book Number 0-309-08450-4

Additional copies of this report are available from National Academy Press, 2101 Constitution Avenue, N.W., Washington, DC 20418

Call (800) 624-6242 or (202) 334-3313 (in the Washington metropolitan area)

This report is also available online at **http://www.nap.edu**

Printed in the United States of America

Copyright 2002 by the National Academy of Sciences. All rights reserved.

Suggested citation: National Research Council (2002) *Leveraging Longitudinal Data in Developing Countries: Report of a Workshop.* Workshop on Leveraging Longitudinal Data in Developing Countries Committee, Committee on Population. Valerie L. Durrant and Jane Menken, editors. Division of Behavioral and Social Sciences and Education. Washington, DC: National Academy Press.

THE NATIONAL ACADEMIES

National Academy of Sciences
National Academy of Engineering
Institute of Medicine
National Research Council

The **National Academy of Sciences** is a private, nonprofit, self-perpetuating society of distinguished scholars engaged in scientific and engineering research, dedicated to the furtherance of science and technology and to their use for the general welfare. Upon the authority of the charter granted to it by the Congress in 1863, the Academy has a mandate that requires it to advise the federal government on scientific and technical matters. Dr. Bruce M. Alberts is president of the National Academy of Sciences.

The **National Academy of Engineering** was established in 1964, under the charter of the National Academy of Sciences, as a parallel organization of outstanding engineers. It is autonomous in its administration and in the selection of its members, sharing with the National Academy of Sciences the responsibility for advising the federal government. The National Academy of Engineering also sponsors engineering programs aimed at meeting national needs, encourages education and research, and recognizes the superior achievements of engineers. Dr. Wm. A. Wulf is president of the National Academy of Engineering.

The **Institute of Medicine** was established in 1970 by the National Academy of Sciences to secure the services of eminent members of appropriate professions in the examination of policy matters pertaining to the health of the public. The Institute acts under the responsibility given to the National Academy of Sciences by its congressional charter to be an adviser to the federal government and, upon its own initiative, to identify issues of medical care, research, and education. Dr. Kenneth I. Shine is president of the Institute of Medicine.

The **National Research Council** was organized by the National Academy of Sciences in 1916 to associate the broad community of science and technology with the Academy's purposes of furthering knowledge and advising the federal government. Functioning in accordance with general policies determined by the Academy, the Council has become the principal operating agency of both the National Academy of Sciences and the National Academy of Engineering in providing services to the government, the public, and the scientific and engineering communities. The Council is administered jointly by both Academies and the Institute of Medicine. Dr. Bruce M. Alberts and Dr. Wm. A. Wulf are chairman and vice chairman, respectively, of the National Research Council.

WORKSHOP ON LEVERAGING LONGITUDINAL DATA IN DEVELOPING COUNTRIES COMMITTEE

Jane Menken (*Chair*), Institute of Behavioral Sciences, University of Colorado, Boulder
Stan Becker, Bloomberg School of Public Health, Johns Hopkins University
Sam Clark, Population Studies Center, University of Pennsylvania
Ronald H. Gray, Bloomberg School of Public Health, Johns Hopkins University
Allan G. Hill, Department of Population and International Health, Harvard School of Public Health
David I. Kertzer, Department of Anthropology, Brown University
James F. Phillips, Population Council, New York, NY
Barry Popkin, Carolina Population Center, University of North Carolina, Chapel Hill

Valerie L. Durrant, *Study Director*
Barney Cohen, *Director*, Committee on Population
Brian Tobachnick, *Project Assistant* (until August 2001)
Christine Chen, *Project Assistant*
Ana-Maria Ignat, *Project Assistant* (since October 2001)

COMMITTEE ON POPULATION

Jane Menken *(Chair),* Institute of Behavioral Sciences, University of Colorado, Boulder
Ellen Brennan-Galvin, Woodrow Wilson Center for International Scholars, Washington, DC
Janet Currie, Department of Economics, University of California, Los Angeles
John N. Hobcraft, Population Investigation Committee, London School of Economics
Charles B. Keely, Institute for the Study of International Migration, Georgetown University
David I. Kertzer, Department of Anthropology, Brown University
David A. Lam, Population Studies Center, University of Michigan, Ann Arbor
Cynthia B. Lloyd, The Population Council, New York
W. Henry Mosley, Department of Population and Family Health Sciences, Johns Hopkins University
Alberto Palloni, Center for Demography and Ecology, University of Wisconsin, Madison
James W. Vaupel, Max Planck Institute for Demographic Research, Rostock, Germany
Kenneth W. Wachter, Department of Demography, University of California, Berkeley
Linda J. Waite, Population Research Center, University of Chicago

Barney Cohen, *Director*

Preface

This report summarizes the presentations and discussion at the Workshop on Leveraging Longitudinal Data in Developing Countries, organized by the Committee on Population of the National Research Council (NRC), in Washington, D.C., June 21-22, 2001.

The workshop would not have been possible without the efforts of several people, some of whom deserve specific mention. The committee is very grateful to Carolyn Makinson of the Andrew W. Mellon Foundation for her persistent interest in this topic that led to the workshop and for her intellectual input during the development of the workshop. Committee on Population member W. Henry Mosley participated in the planning meeting for the workshop. We appreciate his many intellectual contributions, particularly on the history of longitudinal community studies. Funding for the workshop was provided by the Andrew W. Mellon Foundation, U.S. Agency for International Development, and the William and Flora Hewlett Foundation. Fred Binka, Sam Clark, James F. Phillips, and Stephen Tollman participated in an initial planning meeting that helped to shape the workshop before the workshop committee was named.

The staff at the NRC managed the workshop and made it all possible. Valerie L. Durrant, study director, provided a constant intellectual and managerial presence for the project, from the organization of the workshop to the publication of this report. Brian Tobachnick and Ana-Maria Ignat, project assistants, coordinated the travel and arrangements for the workshop and provided administrative support throughout the project. Sabra Bissette Ledent edited the report, and Yvonne Wise managed the manuscript through the publication process. The work was carried out under the general direction of the director of the Committee on Population, Barney Cohen.

The report that constitutes Part I of this volume has been reviewed in draft form by individuals chosen for their diverse perspectives and technical expertise, in accordance with procedures approved by the Report Review Committee of the NRC. The purpose of this independent review is to provide candid and critical comments that will assist the institution in making the published report as sound as possible and to ensure that the report meets institutional standards for objectivity, evidence, and responsiveness to the study charge. The review comments and draft manuscript remain confidential to protect the integrity of the deliberative process.

We thank the following individuals for their participation in the review of this report: John Haaga, Population Reference Bureau, Washington, D.C.; Frank Stafford, Institute for Social Research, University of Michigan; and John Wyon, Harvard School of Public Health (emeritus).

Although the reviewers listed above have provided many constructive comments and suggestions, they were not asked to endorse the final draft of the report before its release. The review of this report was overseen by Julie DaVanzo, RAND. Appointed by the NRC, she was responsible for making certain that an independent examination of this report was carried out in accordance with institutional procedures and that all review comments were carefully considered. Responsibility for the final content of this report rests entirely with the authoring committee and the institution.

Also, we thank the reviewers of the two commissioned papers that constitute Part II of this volume: Linda Adair, University of North Carolina; Stan Becker, Johns Hopkins University; Sam Clark, University of Pennsylvania; Ruth Macklin, Albert Einstein College of Medicine; and Duncan Thomas, RAND.

Jane Menken
Chair, Committee on Population

Contents

PART I REPORT   1

Leveraging Longitudinal Data in Developing Countries   3
    Introduction, 3
    Benefits of Longitudinal Data, 8
    Comparison of Different Approaches to Longitudinal Data, 13
    Challenges to Longitudinal Research, 23
    Strengthening Longitudinal Efforts, 32
    Conclusion, 47
    References, 48

PART II PAPERS   53

Demographic Analysis of Community, Cohort, and Panel Data
from Low-Income Countries: Methodological Issues   55
    Andrew Foster

Overview of Ethical Issues in Collecting Data in Developing
Countries, with Special Reference to Longitudinal Designs   75
    Richard A. Cash and Tracy L. Rabin

APPENDIXES

A Workshop Agenda   97
B Workshop Participants   101

PART I

REPORT

Leveraging Longitudinal Data in Developing Countries

INTRODUCTION

Longitudinal data collection and analysis are critical to social, demographic, and health research, policy, and practice. They are regularly used to address questions of demographic and health trends, policy and program evaluation, and causality. Panel studies, cohort studies, and longitudinal community studies have proved particularly important in developing countries that lack vital registration systems and comprehensive sources of information on the demographic and health situation of their populations. Research using data from such studies has led to scientific advances and improvements in the well-being of individuals in developing countries. Yet questions remain about the usefulness of these studies relative to their expense (and relative to cross-sectional surveys) and about the appropriate choice of alternative longitudinal strategies in different contexts.

For these reasons, the Committee on Population convened a workshop to examine the comparative strengths and weaknesses of various longitudinal approaches in addressing demographic and health questions in developing countries and to consider ways to strengthen longitudinal data collection and analysis. This report summarizes the discussion and opinions voiced at that workshop.

The term *longitudinal studies* encompasses all studies in which a defined population is interviewed over an extended period of time. This workshop focused only on studies that gather information from the same respondents in two or more waves of data collection.[1] Therefore, the discussion in this report may not be applicable to longitudinal studies that select respondents in each wave from a common sample pool (such as a community or other sampling unit) rather than follow the same individuals.

The workshop distinguished three types of longitudinal studies. *Panel studies*[2] are usually broad-based in sample and topical coverage, and frequently use the household as the sampling unit. In that case, information is collected from all or a sample of members of the selected households. *Cohort studies,* a subset of panel studies, follow a sample of people selected on the basis of a common age- or time-specific characteristic (such as birth year, age, or class membership). In some cases, the households to which cohort members belong may be included in the study. *Longitudinal community studies,* also known as *population laboratories* or *demographic surveillance studies,* systematically collect data (generally on fertility, mortality, and in- and out-migration) from *all* individuals (at least all individuals of interest in all households) in geographically demarcated communities. Such studies usually collect data at more frequent intervals than cohort or panel studies, although on a smaller range of topics. The most important distinction, however, relates to the focus of these studies on the community: data are collected from individuals, but the actual unit of observation is the community. Thus in general new people enter the sample as they move into the community, but those who leave the community are not followed.

Background

Information on population and health issues in developing countries during the first half of the 20th century was based on the few censuses that included relevant questions and on a few intensive longitudinal studies. Well-known examples of these studies include the Instituto de Nutrición de Centro América y Panamá (INCAP), which addressed child nutrition in Guatemala, (for a review, see Scrimshaw and Guzman, 1997) and the

---

[1]A paper by Andrew Foster presented at the workshop and reproduced in Part II explores other longitudinal designs.

[2]Barry Popkin presented definitions of the three types of longitudinal studies considered at the workshop.

Khanna study of health and fertility in India (Wyon, 1997; Wyon and Gordon, 1971).

Beginning in the 1960s, individual research institutions initiated multicountry programs of household surveys that greatly expanded the availability of developing country demographic and health information. These programs, which included the Knowledge, Attitude, and Practice (KAP) surveys on contraception (in the 1960s and 1970s), the World Fertility Surveys (1972 -1984), the Demographic and Health Surveys (DHS, which began in 1984 and continues today), and other survey series sponsored by individual research institutions, generally provide nationally representative, widely accessible, and comprehensive data.

Most of these efforts were cross-sectional (data were collected at only one point in time) and focused on the fertility and health status of women and children. Capitalizing on the explicit goal to develop comparable information for a wide range of countries over time, researchers currently use these data widely. The data have proven especially useful for cross-national comparisons. The coverage of household surveys has increased to the point where, by mid-2001, the DHS database alone contained over 100 datasets for 68 countries. Increased general use of DHS (and other) data can be credited to the development of standard recode files. Moreover, the speed with which survey data are made available to the public and with which analytic studies are conducted and their results published has increased remarkably. The DHS surveys are currently available on the World Wide Web.

The number of longitudinal community studies also has increased dramatically (Kahn and Tollman, 1998). A few of these studies have their roots in the 1950s and 1960s such as the Matlab study in Bangladesh (Aziz and Mosley, 1997); the Khanna (Wyon and Gordon, 1971), Singur (Garenne and Koumans, 1997), and Narangwal (Taylor and De Sweemer, 1997) studies in India; The Medical Social Research Project at Lulliani in Pakistan (Garenne and Koumans, 1997); and the ORSTOM (l'Institut Français de Recherche Scientifique pour le Développement en Coopération) study in rural Senegal (Garenne and Cantrelle, 1997; Garenne and Cantrelle, 2001; Cantrelle, 1969). However, most began in the late 1980s and 1990s (Alderman et al., 2001; Mosley, 1989). Many of these studies were undertaken to evaluate specific interventions such as family planning programs, vaccine-trials, or treatments for specific diseases (Das Gupta et al., 1997). However, research inquiries were often broadened beyond their original intent, extending the life of the study long after the original questions were addressed and enhancing their value for other researchers. Some critics believe these studies, which are time-consuming and expensive because of the repeated collection of data at short intervals, have resulted in findings and publications that may be too limited to justify adding new sites and, in some cases, continuing existing efforts.

The current situation is therefore one in which the number of studies of various types (including but not limited to longitudinal studies and cross-sectional surveys) is large and growing. Yet, at the same time, policy makers are increasingly demanding rapid analysis and policy-relevant findings, and new analytical tools are expanding the ways in which data from studies of different types can be used. In addition, an increasing number of institutions and data collection sites are requesting access to limited funds in circumstances of growing competition and often more costly research environments.

Purpose of the Workshop

In this context, the Committee on Population convened a Workshop on Leveraging Longitudinal Data in Developing Countries in Washington, D.C., in June 2001. The primary goals of the workshop were to examine the comparative strengths and weaknesses of several longitudinal approaches in addressing demographic and health questions in developing countries and to consider ways to strengthen longitudinal data collection and analysis. Workshop participants addressed a wide range of scientific, practical, and strategic issues, concentrating on longitudinal community studies, panel studies, and cohort studies. Africa received special emphasis for two reasons: (1) the ongoing information crisis in the region and (2) the interest of funding agencies in evaluating the potential of expanded investment in longitudinal studies for addressing issues currently crucial to the region.

The intention of the Committee on Population was to provide an arena for discussion among researchers with diverse topical interests, disciplinary backgrounds, experience with longitudinal methods and approaches, and motivations for conducting longitudinal research; it was not to make recommendations about the best longitudinal approaches for various research questions or in various settings. This report provides a summary of the invited presentations and short papers, the discussants' comments, and the general discussion. Two commissioned papers are reproduced in Part II of this report. The technical discussion ranged broadly from comparison of the approaches themselves, to examples of longitudinal studies, to data collection and data management issues, to the relevant innovations in computer science. It also covered additional important and diverse issues, including ethics, collaboration and networking across studies, funding mechanisms, data sharing, capacity building, and researcher/participant/community relations. The workshop agenda is in Appendix A and a list of participants is presented in Appendix B.

At this point, it is important to clarify what topics were *not* covered at the workshop and therefore are not covered in this report. To maximize the time devoted to comparing longitudinal approaches, workshop participants did not address topics related to cross-sectional data, including a comparison of longitudinal and cross-sectional approaches, and to techniques such as synthetic cohort analysis and retrospective data, which can be used with cross-sectional data to simulate longitudinal data. Other aspects of collecting and analyzing longitudinal data also were beyond the scope of the workshop. Relevant topics that were not adequately addressed include: tracking respondents (methods or costs); dealing with "split-offs" or changes in the sample produced when members of a household in the study leave the household (such as adult children moving out to establish their own household and separations and divorces); "refreshing" a sample (adding new respondents for those who drop out); changing survey questions if a better approach is developed over the course of a study; deciding on the optimal interval between interviews; analyzing longitudinal data (strategies and techniques); keeping data users informed about features of the data (e.g., if oddities or errors are discovered in the data); and including retrospective data collection in the first wave of a study.

Organization of the Report

This report has two parts. Part I includes an overview of the presentations and discussion at the workshop presented in four sections. The first section considers the benefits of longitudinal data in general. The section that follows compares the advantages and disadvantages of panel studies, cohort studies, and longitudinal community studies and presents considerations for determining the best approach. The third section examines challenges to longitudinal research, highlighting those associated with funding, relationships with respondents, attrition and population change, research biases, and ethics. The final section explores several ways in which longitudinal research efforts can be strengthened to increase returns to researchers, respondents, policy makers, and the scientific community. Part II of the report includes two of the papers presented at the workshop. The first paper, by Andrew Foster, compares panel, cohort, and longitudinal community studies in low-income countries from a methodological perspective. The second paper, by Richard A. Cash and Tracy L. Rabin, presents an overview of ethical issues in developing country research with special reference to longitudinal data. The workshop agenda and the list of workshop participants are included as appendixes.

BENEFITS OF LONGITUDINAL DATA

Throughout the workshop discussion, participants noted the strengths of longitudinal research, even though identifying the advantages of longitudinal studies relative to those of cross-sectional studies was not an objective of the workshop.[3] Yet while mentioning the virtues of longitudinal efforts, they continually noted that the use of longitudinal data and the specific approach adopted depend on the research question at hand. For many time-dependent research questions, synthetic cohorts (using cross-sectional data in a way that builds on age groups, representing birth cohorts, to examine how events of interest change over time) or retrospective data from cross-sectional studies may be equally or even more useful and have the additional benefits of lower cost and time intensity. Even when the research question demands longitudinal data, without sufficient time and money for follow-up, longitudinal efforts may be futile.

The benefits of longitudinal research discussed at the workshop can be grouped into two general areas: (1) contributing to scientific knowledge and (2) promoting careful research practices and designs.

Contributing to Scientific Knowledge

Workshop participants suggested that longitudinal research contributes to understanding causal relationships by collecting more accurate and detailed information on the timing and sequence of various events than might otherwise be obtainable. It also seems to permit greater accuracy by[4] :

---

[3]This section is based on presentations by Linda Adair, Ties Boerma, Andrew Foster, Barry Popkin, and Stephen Tollman.

[4]This section is based on the presentation by Andrew Foster.

- examining changes in various behaviors and related events over time with observations close to the time of the change or event
- addressing selectivity problems (such as the background characteristics of respondents that may confound the relationship between the variables of interest) in statistical analyses with fewer assumptions
- studying programs or sources of change in which there are lags between the introduction of an intervention and its possible effects.

The advantage of longitudinal data relates specifically to researchers' ability to look at change (e.g., before and after differences) for a given individual while, in the process, netting out the effect of (unobserved) characteristics of the individual that do not change over time. With cross-sectional data, researchers compare different individuals at a point in time and must be concerned that differences along the dimension of interest might be due to other (unobserved) differences among individuals.

Longitudinal research of various types has led to a substantial body of scientific and policy-relevant findings. Scientifically, the availability of longitudinal data has allowed researchers to better understand human, social, and economic development processes, to test more dynamic and complex theories of social and health behaviors, and to refine their understanding of causal relationships. Studies have illuminated the health, social, and economic needs of individuals, communities, or subgroups of populations; evaluated the effectiveness of a range of programs and interventions; and enabled policy makers and planners to set priorities based on evidence. Table 1 pulls together some specific examples of study findings that were mentioned at the workshop. In the opinion of several workshop participants, the contributions of longitudinal research to science have been much greater than those to policy to date.

The benefits of longitudinal research can become clearer when research is related to a particular topic, and Ties Boerma did just that in his presentation on the human immunodeficiency virus (HIV) and other sexually transmitted diseases (STDs). Through longitudinal studies of HIV/STDs, researchers now better understand the complex interactions among the biomedical and social determinants of HIV and other STDs. These studies include investigations of the trends and determinants of HIV infection; the impacts of HIV and other STDs on fertility, adult and child mortality, and population size; and the interactions among demographic factors, such as age and migration, and socioeconomic, cultural, and biological factors in the acquired immunodeficiency syndrome (AIDS) epidemic. Longitudi-

TABLE 1 Examples of Lessons Learned from Longitudinal Data Presented at the Workshop

Study	Findings
Cohort Studies	
INCAP (Guatemala)	Inter-relationships of diet, nutritional status, and infection[a] (particularly the sequencing[b])
Khanna (India)	Breastfeeding alone is insufficient to supply the calories needed by infants six months and older; supplementary foods are required for infants to fight common intestinal and respiratory diseases
Cebu (Philippines)	Long-term effects of stunting[c]
INCAP	Economic, health, and developmental effects of key developmental patterns[d]
	Rationale for multipurpose child care focus in development
	Fetal programming (Barker hypothesis): adult health outcomes affected by prenatal and early postnatal environment
Panel Studies	
IFLS (Indonesia)	Household adjustments to macroeconomic shocks
CHNS (China)[e]	Increased malnutrition among rural poor (leading to government policies to lower food prices and initiate anti-poverty efforts)
RLMS (Russia)[f]	Privatization's effect on poverty: major expansion of long-term poor
	Increased gender and economic inequality
Longitudinal Community Studies	
Rufiji, Tanzania	Location of health facilities, use of health services, and infant and child health
	Mortality burden of malaria (especially for children)
Bandim, Guinea-Bissau	Risks of Diptheria, Pertussis, and Tetanus (DPT) vaccination for young infants (less than 3 months old); importance of when vaccinations are administered
Matlab, Bangladesh	DPT vaccinations among children between three and five months and decreased mortality

TABLE 1 Continued

Study	Findings
Manhica, Mozambique	Rapid increase in mortality of children under age five in year 2000 (possibly as a consequence of the stress of the January-February 2000 floods)
Ifakara, Tanzania	Insecticide treated bednets and reduced under-five mortality

SOURCE: Based on presentations by Linda Adair, Barry Popkin, Stephen Tollman, and INDEPTH information.

NOTE: This table reflects the experience of particular workshop presenters rather than a comprehensive or systematic picture of the field. It should be viewed as illustratious of the range of rich findings generated through longitudinal analyses of various types. INCAP=Instituto de Nutrición de Centro América y Panamá; IFLS=Indonesian Family Life Survey; CHNS=China Health and Nutrition Survey; RLMS=Russian Longitudinal Monitoring Survey.

[a] Martorell et al. (1990).
[b] Ramakrishnan (1999a); Schroeder et al. (1999); Martorell (1995); Martorell et al. (1995); Ruel et al. (1995).
[c] Mendez and Adair (1999) and Adair and Guilkey (1997).
[d] Ramakrishnan et al. (1999b).
[e] Guo et al. (2000) and Bell et al. (2001).
[f] Lokshin et al. (2000); Lokshin and Popkin (1999); Popkin and Mroz (1995).

nal studies have provided some information (based on verbal autopsies) on the impact of AIDS on mortality. Longitudinal studies undertaken to evaluate interventions aimed at reducing HIV infection (including community trials) have yielded important information on HIV and sexually transmitted diseases.

The future of HIV/STDs research is likely to continue to be dominated by intervention studies (albeit focused on various aspects of transmission, prevention, and cure). Boerma foresees that more gains in knowledge about HIV/STDs and related population and health issues will require more studies using population-based samples (as opposed to clinic clients or other ad hoc groups) and larger comparison populations. He expects to see more studies that examine HIV/STDs and other aspects of health in a broader perspective and over a longer-term than the current short-term intervention studies. A challenge lies in how to develop ways to overcome the short-lived nature of intervention studies and establish long-term population cohort studies.

Promoting Careful Research Practice and Designs

Another major contribution of longitudinal research, in addition to the many and diverse specific findings it has yielded, is related to the iterative and dynamic processes of inquiry these studies require and the careful research practices and designs they promote. The importance of this kind of contribution was a key theme of presentations by Barry Popkin, Stephen Tollman, and Robert Willis.

Barry Popkin traced the historical evolution of cohort and household panel studies from the very focused studies of specific topics prior to the 1970s, particularly in the field of public health, to the multipurpose and broad-based studies of today. He argued that six changes in approach have improved the scientific and policy impact of these types of longitudinal surveys:

(1) the shift from single purpose to multipurpose surveys.
(2) the shift from retrospective to prospective data.
(3) the shift from individual-level data collection to multilevel data collection, especially community data collected concurrently with individual and household data.
(4) the integration of qualitative work.
(5) the addition of a biomedical perspective to social science work. and
(6) the addition of natural sciences and ecology in the mid-1990s.

Stephen Tollman, in discussing the contributions of longitudinal community studies to science and policy, pointed to specific findings (see Table 1) that have emerged from longitudinal community studies and the overall process of serendipity and feedback that makes a critical contribution to such studies. Drawing on experience from the INDEPTH network (an International Network of field sites with continuous Demographic Evaluation of Populations and Their Health in developing countries), he emphasized the long-term research benefits facilitated by two other key features of longitudinal community studies: (1) the engagement with the community and (2) the development of research infrastructure.

Finally, in a presentation on the lessons learned from the long history of longitudinal studies in the United States, Robert Willis stressed the importance of sound and appropriate designs using the Health and Retirement Study (HRS) and the Asset and Health Dynamics of the Oldest Old (AHEAD) study as examples. These two studies, developed as cohort studies to examine effects of aging on the health and economic well-being of Americans and related policy issues, began with two different age groups but were merged in 1993 and expanded in 1998 with the addition of new cohorts (of the same age as the original cohorts were at entry). HRS designers switched to a steady state design in order to present an ongoing picture of the U.S. population over age 50. Their goals were to promote better understanding of the effects of aging on the well-being of individuals and any changes in those effects that may occur over time, and to improve the capacity of researchers to analyze the effects of social and policy changes as they occur in the future (Willis, 1999).

COMPARISON OF DIFFERENT APPROACHES TO LONGITUDINAL DATA

Panel studies, cohort studies, and longitudinal community studies are, of course, not equivalent in their objectives or their ability to answer specific social sciences questions. As noted earlier, the research question and the goals of the research project, along with context, funding, and other considerations, must be taken into account in determining the best study approach.

Workshop participants raised some of the issues that should be considered in determining the best longitudinal approach for a particular study. The issues include the following eight items:

1. What is the research question? How can the question best be answered? What types of indicators and measures and what frequency of observation are required to answer the research question (and are these particularly amenable to a certain longitudinal approach)?

2. What is the context for the study? (What other data on the study area are available? What data are needed? What burden, if any, will the study pose for respondents? Could other studies or activities in the area pose the risk of contamination?)

3. Does the study population need to be representative to a larger population (such as a country or region)?

4. Is there adequate spatial and temporal variability in the main independent and outcome measures?

5. Which is more important to address the research question properly: geographical coverage of a particular area or sample size?

6. What are the main purposes of the undertaking and future plans (e.g., scientific research, capacity building, local investment and infrastructure)?

7. For topic or sample coverage, which is more important—scope or depth?

8. What ethical considerations are most relevant for the intended research goals?

Andrew Foster compared the strengths and weaknesses of panel, cohort, and longitudinal comparative studies for three purposes: measurement/description, program evaluation, and structural analysis (hypothesis testing and statistical modeling). A summary based on his presentation and further elaboration by others at the workshop is presented in Table 2.

For **measurement**, or description, of demographic and health processes or patterns, the major differences among the three approaches stem primarily from the differences in the target populations. Panel studies generally cover a broad population, whereas cohort and longitudinal communities focus on specific subpopulations (based on a common characteristic for cohort studies and on a specific community or geographic area for longitudinal community studies). These differences affect the degree to which findings from a longitudinal study can be generalized to other areas of the country and the extent to which inferences can be made. In addition, the greater depth and breadth of data collected in most panel and cohort studies enhances their analysis options, whereas most longitudinal community studies typically measure selected (but limited) events in much greater detail and have larger sample sizes, enabling better observation of many rare events.

As for **program evaluation**, the representativeness of the study population to the general population is less salient than other characteristics in determining the suitability of each approach for assessing the impact of community-level interventions. Evaluation is especially sensitive to changes in the study population, so continuity of the sample across time is more important than whether the sample is representative of a larger population.

Thus, longitudinal community studies, which deliberately follow all members of the community, are ideal for assessing program impacts. Panel and cohort studies may be affected by losses in the study population (such as through migration or other changes in household composition) unless they try to follow respondents who move. Cohort studies are further limited by the selection of the sample according to characteristics that may or may not be appropriate for evaluating the program of interest.

On the other hand, longitudinal studies that are located in many communities often take advantage of the community variation (e.g., use community characteristics to achieve statistical identification). Studies that focus on only one community (or a few communities), including most longitudinal community studies, cannot do this.

Differences in the heterogeneity of the sample between longitudinal community studies, on the one hand, and panel and cohort studies, on the other, create different opportunities for program evaluation. Because longitudinal community studies are often tied directly to interventions in specific areas (with control groups in other areas), it is not necessary to have a lot of variation within the sample; the interesting variation is imposed through the experimental design. By contrast, panel and cohort studies, with their broad geographic coverage, require a heterogeneous sample in order to produce variability in outcomes of interest to study.

Under opportune circumstances, however, carefully situated and planned evaluations can be effectively conducted with panel and cohort studies, and they are likely to require less investment than longitudinal community studies and to inspire fewer concerns about the generalizability of findings and the aspects of the study community that may influence findings.

The three approaches differ least in their usefulness for **structural analysis.** The techniques used in these analyses and their data requirements vary greatly, so that the variation within a longitudinal approach is often greater than the variation across different approaches.

In terms of enhancing community participation and strengthening local research capacity, longitudinal community studies outperform the other longitudinal approaches. The primary objectives of longitudinal community studies extend beyond their potential to advance immediate knowledge. Specifically, enhancing community participation and strengthening local research infrastructures are typically key components of these studies, especially when controlled trials are to be undertaken. The involvement of local communities and capacity strengthening may be, and often are, im-

TABLE 2 Session 1—Comparisons of Panel Cohort and Longitudinal Community Studies Discussed at the Workshop

	Panel Studies
General definition	Usually broad-based in sample and topical coverage. Household is frequently the sampling unit.
Capacity strengthening	Generally work with established institutions and researchers in country
	Offer temporary jobs, mostly for data collecting, data entry, and coding
	Generally work with researchers and policy makers at the national level
Ethical concerns	Protecting confidentiality of individual respondents, particularly when sharing data
	Obligations to respondents to provide results that may be produced from the data years after data collection

Cohort Studies	Longitudinal Community Studies
Subset of panel studies. Follow a sample of people selected on the basis of a common age- or time-specific characteristic (such as birth year, age, or class membership). May include information on households to which cohort members belong.	Systematically collect data (generally on fertility, mortality, and in- and out-migration) from *all* individuals in geographically demarcated communities. Data are generally collected at more frequent intervals than for cohort or panel studies, although on a smaller range of topics. Communities are the primary unit of observation (though data come from individuals). Also referred to as *population laboratories* or *demographic surveillance studies*.
Generally work with established institutions and researchers in country	Establish long-term research center at site
Offer temporary jobs, mostly for data collecting, data entry, and coding	Offer range of employment opportunities
Generally work with researchers and policy makers at the national level	Generally work with researchers and policy makers at the local (community) level
Protecting confidentiality of individual respondents, particularly when sharing data	Protecting confidentiality of individual respondents
Obligations to respondents to provide results that may be produced from the data years after data collection	Protecting confidentiality of the communities in which respondents live (especially for small-area studies)
	Obligations to respondents to provide results that may be produced from the data years after data collection

Continued

TABLE 2 Session 1—Continued

Comparison for different research goals:
Panel Studies

Research goal: measurement/description.
Measuring and describing patterns of demographic change (computation of vital rates and other aspects of individual and household welfare) and changes in these measures and patterns over time.

Advantages	Most likely to be representative of large-area population
	Greater depth and breadth in socioeconomic and health measures
Disadvantages	Need to refresh panels to remain representative over time
	Often have few observations of rare events

Cohort Studies	Longitudinal Community Studies
Representative of group born in a particular cohort	Provides detailed information on specific community(ies)
Greater depth and breadth in socioeconomic and health measures	Decrease the costs and increase the quality of longitudinal data collection in specific community(ies) by establishing research infrastructure
	Allows precise estimation of mortality through larger (person-year) samples and greater focus on rare events
	Utilize greater periodicity of measurement
Not representative of or generalizable to general population	Not necessarily representative of other communities; no way to obtain statistical estimate of cross-community variability to derive estimates.
Often have few observations of rare events	Outmigrants excluded from subsequent surveys

Continued

TABLE 2 Session 1—Continued

Panel Studies

Research goal: program evaluation
Obtaining estimates of program and intervention effectiveness by collecting indicators at two or more points in time before, during, or after program implementation. Often looking at the same individual over time is less important than looking at community effects, or comparisons between individuals or groups of similar ages at time 1 and time 2.

Advantages	Capture greater spatial variability.
	Allow evaluations of programs focused on geographic areas to control for endogeneity of program placement.
Disadvantages	Significant changes in the sample will inhibit ability to yield good estimates.
	May have insufficient sample sizes in communities where interventions are placed to study program impacts.

Research goal: structural analysis
Uncovering the mechanisms underlying observed outcomes; hypothesis testing.

Advantages	Generally have a broad range of variables.
	Useful in looking at short- and long-term outcomes (depending on length of study).
	Conducive to large, representative samples.

Cohort Studies	Longitudinal Community Studies
Capture greater spatial variability.	Ideal for program evaluation at the community level because of deliberate tracking of entrants, leavers, and relevant behaviors of all members that can be compared at any given points in time.
Allow evaluations of programs focused. on geographic areas to control for endogeneity of program placement.	
Significant changes in the sample will inhibit ability to yield good estimates.	Limited geographic coverage, raises concerns about • spatially autocorrelated variables • logistical considerations surrounding placement of program villages • generalizability of findings.
Because of age-specific nature of sample, any program effects related to age are more difficult to evaluate using cohort data (unless the intervention is specific to the cohort being studied).	
Data can become dated or useless if changes in the social and political environment change the nature of the cohort of interest (e.g, a change in Medicare laws will affect studies of the health of the elderly).	Limited range of variables may impede ability to control for many confounding factors (though several studies include a broad range of variables).
Generally have a broad range of variables.	Because of the population coverage, generally include information necessary for a panel study and a cohort study—opening the possibility for a range of longitudinal studies and approaches.
Useful in looking at short- and long-term outcomes (depending on length of study).	
Useful for understanding life events and cumulative and lifelong exposures to various effects.	Useful in looking at short- and long-term outcomes (depending on length of study).

Continued

TABLE 2 Session 1—Continued

	Panel Studies
Disadvantages	Attrition can compromise representativeness and estimates
	Often miss rare events

SOURCE: Based on presentations by Andrew Foster, Linda Adair, Jim Phillips, Duncan Thomas, and Barry Popkin and on comments by participants in the workshop.

portant elements of panel and cohort studies, but they are generally not explicit objectives of these approaches. Although some capacity strengthening does accompany panel and cohort studies, especially for the in-country collaborating institutions and for studies connected to U.S. institutions in the past decade through the Fogarty International Center (FIC) at the U.S. National Institutes of Health (discussed later in this report), comprehensive approaches to capacity strengthening and community participation have been concentrated within longitudinal community studies.

At several points in the discussion, workshop participants expressed the sentiment that, though particular methods of longitudinal data collection and analysis may better suit particular research questions, the potential for knowledge multiplies when different longitudinal approaches are used in conjunction (this point is discussed later in the section on "Strengthening Longitudinal Efforts").

Cohort Studies	Longitudinal Community Studies
	Good at capturing rare events because of the population coverage
	Maximize ability to incorporate serendipity and feedback because of regular intervals of data collection and research infrastructure
Attrition can compromise representativeness and estimates	Attrition can compromise representativeness and estimates.
Often miss rare events	Nonrepresentative beyond community in which data are collected
Problems with estimation: endogeneity (including altered behavior in response to various factors of interest) and difficulty identifying age and period effects	Often include small sample sizes
	Randomized at the community level, and so introduces statistical inefficiency

CHALLENGES TO LONGITUDINAL RESEARCH

Despite the benefits of longitudinal research for science and policy, some challenges must be addressed. Good longitudinal efforts tend to be resource-intensive in funding requirements, design and planning, research subject and community participation, and investigators' investment of time. Institutional (or researcher) continuity is needed to provide the memory and direction for long, complex studies, particularly those requiring several years of observations to generate findings. Additional problems relate to the mobility of respondents and change in the communities under study, as well as the ethical considerations unique to this type of research. Five challenges to working with longitudinal data are described in this section: (1) funding, (2) relationships with communities and respondents, (3) changes in samples, (4) changes in study protocols, and (5) ethical research practices.

Funding

Researchers face the challenge of obtaining and sustaining investment in their projects over a long period. Because of several issues related to the costs, competition for funding, and time requirements of longitudinal data, researchers find it difficult to determine when to terminate, scale back, or maintain or increase research efforts. Workshop participants recognized the possibility that continuing data collection in one site may have diminishing returns compared with starting over in another site, especially when sample attrition or other sample changes affect the representativeness of the sample. However, the cost-effectiveness and other strategic interests associated with continuing, moving, or ending studies was not a topic addressed by the workshop.

Longitudinal studies are more expensive than cross-sectional studies with similar sample size and design (though not necessarily more expensive than repeated cross-sections with the same number of waves). Data are collected repeatedly (at least twice) from respondents. To maintain the integrity of the study, respondents must be tracked over time. Throughout the process, the huge amounts of data generated must be managed and analyzed by project staff.

As the number of longitudinal study sites has grown, the competition for funds has increased. This competition affects both researchers' abilities to start-up new studies and the long-term sustainability of existing sites. Because of the time requirements and the long-term nature of longitudinal studies, researchers often must rely on limited substantive results for continued funding. With the demands of data collection and management and proposal writing, researchers frequently find themselves lacking the time and resources to analyze the data. Studies therefore often fail, in the eyes of many, to achieve their research potential.

It also takes years for longitudinal studies to produce substantive results. A lag between study initiation and study results is often expected because longitudinal studies are intended to look at trends and long-term effects. The long germination period required by many longitudinal studies was demonstrated with two examples at the workshop. First, Barry Popkin and Linda Adair cited David Barker's work on the effects of the prenatal and early-natal environment on adult health outcomes as an example of how significant returns to longitudinal studies may emerge years after study initiation (Adair et al., 2001; Barker, 1998; Popkin et al., 1996).

Second, Jane Menken presented results from a study in Bangladesh in which she and her colleagues examined the effects of early life characteristics on later survival. They linked detailed information on women collected in the 1976 Determinants of Natural Fertility Study (including health, nonpregnant weight, fertility history, and household socioeconomic status) with survival data from the International Centre for Health and Population Research's Demographic Surveillance System in Matlab, Bangladesh, and demonstrated that the effects of socioeconomic and health status in early adulthood persist over the next 20 years. However, the effects of certain key variables on the odds of dying became statistically significant only after 10 years of follow-up (body mass index), 15 years of follow-up (no schooling), or even later (being Hindu was approaching statistical significance at 20 years of follow-up).

Relationships with Communities and Respondents

All longitudinal studies depend on the cooperation of respondents and their communities for the duration of the study. Yet, the demands on respondents and their communities, and the extent to which they are integrated into the research process, differ with the type of study because of different objectives, study populations, practices, and researcher presence in the community. Generally, the longer the relationship with the community and the greater the demands on the participants, the greater is the need for community participation and perceived returns to participants and communities in the research process.

On the one hand, in two-wave panel studies researchers survey respondents and then survey them again some time later. The demands on the respondents and their communities are minimal, generally limited to sampling and data collection needs. The potential benefits to the respondents and their communities are also limited—to any direct compensation for participation or relevant findings that emerge (if shared with the communities). On the other hand, longitudinal community studies have a strong long-term presence in a specific (generally relatively small) study site, and researchers collect data at regular (and often short) intervals from all households. It is therefore vital that researchers have a good rapport and working relationships with community leaders, respondents, and local professionals throughout the process.

Community participation is crucial in three situations: (1) when sensitive topics are included in the research scope; (2) when studies are concentrated in smaller physical areas; and (3) when research involves multiple revisits or complicated questionnaires or research requirements (such as medical tests or time-use diaries). This point was illustrated by James F. Phillips, who described the process through which a study of female genital mutilation (FGM) was integrated into an ongoing longitudinal community study in Navrongo, Ghana, without disrupting ongoing research efforts. The researchers held many meetings and discussions with community leaders and members over several months about whether and how to add questions on FGM to the survey. With community support, they were able to gather data on FGM without compromising their overall goals or the continuing participation of respondents. In the Navrongo project, community leaders have participated in many aspects of the study.

Another dimension of project-community relations involves the returns to communities and individuals from the research activities. These returns range from direct benefits at the research site (such as employment on the project) to increased knowledge and well-being as the results of the studies filter back to the community through information sharing and new policies and programs. Benefits to the community, while desired by many researchers, generally are achieved only through intentional objectives and strategies.

Changes in the Sample

Study populations and samples change over time, affecting longitudinal research. People are added to the study population through in-migration and births and removed from study populations and samples through out-migration, deaths, and refusals to participate. Current demographic patterns in many developing areas suggest that longitudinal researchers need to be aware of these changes; however, information is often insufficient to allow researchers to anticipate specific changes.

Studies differ in the extent to which they accommodate changes by tracking migrants or refreshing the sample. In Cebu, Philippines entire slums have been razed and the number of communities where respondents live has grown from 33 to over 260 as respondents have dispersed due to migration over 18 years of tracking the original mother-infant cohort. HRS/AHEAD's steady state design, in which new cohorts of those in the youngest age group are added at regular intervals, was incorporated to address losses in the sample (to death) and to keep the sample fresh. The willingness of researchers to track or add respondents and the study objectives affect the need to adjust the study. As mentioned earlier, study areas also differ in the extent to which sample adjustments, tracking, or other efforts prove effective.

Studies differ in their need to address certain population changes. When communities are a key component of the research, studies are more vulnerable to changes, and it is more important to incorporate necessary adjustments. For community-based studies, it is critical to deal with entrants and leavers, though not necessarily through tracking, because the composition of the population in the community (and changes in it) forms the basis for the research. Robert Willis also noted that when context variables (such as community or neighborhood factors) are central aspects of research, sample attrition or change compromises the study if not properly addressed.

Sample attrition is a potential problem for any longitudinal study where researchers want to generalize results. Research has revealed that migrants (respondents who leave) differ in important ways from those who stay. For example, research using the Indonesian Family Life Survey shows that long-distance migrants, short-distance migrants, and nonmigrants differ in educational attainment and earned income levels.[5] Examining longitudinal household surveys from Bolivia, Kenya, and South Africa, Alderman and colleagues (2001) saw significant differences between respondents who were retained and those who were lost in follow-ups. Researchers face additional challenges in areas where migration is circular, with people regularly coming and going from a study area.

Two examples of ways in which to deal with sample changes were presented at the workshop. First, Duncan Thomas described three ways to address change in study samples due to migration:

1. *Track migrants.* Researchers can attempt to follow respondents who have migrated out of the study area and conduct the follow-up survey(s) with respondents who are found.

2. *Adjust the sample.* Researchers can sample a subset of all migrants from the study area and adjust the remaining sample accordingly. Adjustment works best when individuals are the unit of analysis; studies in which households or dwellings are the sampling or identification unit are less amenable to adjustment.

---

[5]This section is based on a presentation by Duncan Thomas.

3. Ignore the changes. Researchers, in some cases, can ignore attrition and population changes.

Thomas reported that efforts between 1997 and 1998 to track migrants in the Indonesian Family Life Survey substantially reduced sample attrition and provided useful information. However, the costs of tracking and interviewing a migrant were about 20 percent more than those for a nonmigrant. Tracking also increases the spread of the study because it entails going to areas that were not originally part of the sample.

Pierre Ngom described his experiences tracking migrants in a study of urban slum residents in Kenya (see Box 1) and pointed out the problems that arise because of changes in the definition of critical units, such as households or dwellings, over time. The costs and difficulties associated with tracking respondents are closely related to the geographic scope of the study. The costs of tracking migrants in the IFLS will be lower than those for a longitudinal community study site because the IFLS has national coverage and therefore study teams at many of the migrant destination sites.

Effects of Changes in Longitudinal Study Protocols

The existence of a research infrastructure (for example, trained interviewers, research center, baseline data) provided by longitudinal studies, especially long-term ones such as longitudinal community studies, may provide an incentive for others to locate independent studies or programs in the area or for researchers to add variables or types of data to their protocols (for example, the existing research infrastructure and baseline information may facilitate evaluation).

Such changes in the study area or research protocol may affect research in two ways: (1) by instigating changes in the study participants and (2) by contaminating the research process. Speaking to the first point, workshop participants raised concerns about whether communities and participants change in reaction to the study—the Hawthorne effect—particularly when multiple revisits to the same respondents or multiple studies in a small area occur. For example, do multiple exposures to survey questions change the reactions of respondents to the questionnaires (e.g., making them more cooperative, more accurate, or more hostile)? Does survey experience stimulate change in respondents' knowledge, attitudes, or behavior by raising awareness of various issues? Survey experience also may affect research

> **BOX 1**
> **Challenges of Longitudinal Community Studies in Urban Slums in Kenya**
>
> In Africa, rapid urbanization, growing poverty and inequity in health outcomes, lack of assessment tools for and knowledge about health and social interventions, and increasing data needs that involve tracking movers in longitudinal studies clearly justify increased longitudinal research in the cities, particularly slums and poor areas. Although longitudinal community studies in Africa have a relatively long history and fill a critical role in collecting demographic and health data, sites have been concentrated in rural areas.
>
> Recently, researchers at the African Population and Health Research Center have initiated a longitudinal community study in an urban slum in Kenya, only the second longitudinal community study conducted in an urban area. Pierre Ngom presented five challenges to conducting longitudinal community studies in urban slums:
>
> 1. Defining residential units, households, and individuals is much more difficult in urban areas than rural areas. Whereas in rural areas households and residential units are easily identifiable and self-contained, urban residents live in units that are impermanent, easily altered, and flexible.
>
> 2. The population is highly mobile. Researchers do not find the same people in the same dwelling unit between two successive interviews.
>
> 3. The right visitation cycle length and residency time thresholds are difficult to determine because of the transient nature of the population and the high numbers of temporary absentees and visitors.
>
> 4. Insecurity and community fatigue (because of a high concentration of research and programs in slum areas) are common characteristics of urban slums. Violence and explosive situations can easily disrupt research and put respondents and researchers in danger. Slum residents are distrustful of researchers.
>
> 5. Software designed for maintaining and using longitudinal data that pertain to rural populations is not easily transferable to urban settings because of different household arrangements and levels of mobility; specific software for urban areas is needed.

findings in evaluation studies if it makes respondents more (or less) accessible to programs—for example, more informed or more open to programs and treatments. These potential influences are not applicable to research based on objective measures such as biomarkers and anthropometry. The data could also become less accurate over time if respondents learn to answer in certain ways to shorten the interview or avoid sensitive questions (for example, respondents may learn that a particular answer to one question leads to a set of additional questions, and in follow-up waves answer the question in such as way as to avoid follow-up questions).

Second, adding new studies, new types of data (such as the collection of biomarkers or a component on FGM), or new programs to a study area may interfere with original study plans. For example, the presence of several concurrent interventions in a study area makes it difficult to demonstrate precise causal processes and effects. Researchers also must grapple with whether to maintain consistency in variables across surveys or change variable measurement if better measures are developed during the course of the study. Community relationships and participation also may be influenced by such changes.

Ethical Research Practices

More rigorous institutional requirements for research on human subjects and greater knowledge about how research practices can affect individuals and communities have led to a heightened emphasis on ethics in demographic and health research. Yet, growing concerns about reducing the costs of longitudinal data collection and increasing public accessibility to the data often come in direct conflict with ethical concerns.

Longitudinal studies are subject to the same ethical considerations as studies in which data are collected at a single-point in time. The three basic principles of ethics in biomedical research—respect for persons, beneficence, and justice—guide most discussions of ethical considerations.[6] These principles encompass broad concerns, including ensuring respondent confidentiality, obtaining informed consent from respondents, and assuring that research benefits outweigh potential risks to respondents (see the paper by Cash and Rabin in Part II).

---

[6]Some researchers, particularly those in the medical sciences, also include a fourth principle (nonmaleficence) of ethics in biomedical research (see the paper by Cash and Rabin in Part II).

Many ethical considerations are compounded in longitudinal data collection. First, identity protection becomes a greater concern because an identification variable must be maintained in the data to link data from the same respondent in subsequent waves, possibly requiring extra measures to protect respondents. Second, the additional variables, attributes, and information contained in the data increase the likelihood that respondents can be identified. This is especially true when studies are concentrated in small physical areas in developing countries. Richard Cash argued that the developing country context has forced researchers to extrapolate the core ethics principles from the individual level to that of the community (further discussed in the Cash and Rabin paper in Part II), which is particularly relevant when researchers return to the same communities over time.

Third, the longer life of longitudinal data generates additional considerations related to researchers' obligations to respondents (for example, providing research results to participants who may move during or after the study or offering treatment for illnesses identified with the research). Obligations to participants are especially important for biomedical research; the concerns may be quite different for social science research in which the studies or interventions pose little risk to participants.

The following ethics-based questions were raised by participants, pointing to the challenges facing researchers who collect and work with longitudinal data:

- Are researchers obliged to track respondents in case of unanticipated results with implications for respondents? If so, for how long?
- What are the time limitations on sharing results with respondents? If results take years to show up, do researchers need to find respondents to share the results with them?
- How do researchers deal with obtaining informed consent from respondents who are minors in one wave of a study and adults in subsequent waves? From whom do researchers need to obtain consent?
- In addition to obtaining consent from respondents for each wave of data, do researchers also need to obtain consent for analysis and research questions that use multiple waves of data? Do researchers need to obtain permission from respondents to use data in ways other than those originally intended?
- Should researchers go back and ask participants for consent for an add-on or unanticipated study? What if returning to get permission may compromise the confidentiality of respondents?

Ethical research practices, particularly related to identification, are especially critical in longitudinal community studies. The geographically specific sites combined with ongoing data collection render longitudinal community studies vulnerable to problems with maintaining the confidentiality and anonymity of respondents. The need to protect the identity of the community itself, particularly if the research topics are sensitive, is another concern for researchers. As awareness of the research spreads, these issues become increasingly challenging. Capacity strengthening efforts also raise concerns about ethics, especially related to what researchers should and can be expected to provide to the community in terms of education, jobs, information, and the like. These concerns were not explored at this workshop.

Common ethical practices in research are evolving to address emerging issues and new technologies. At the U.S. National Institutes of Health, a subject of current debate is whether informed consent should be obtained for third-party subjects. Specifically, should informed consent be solicited from indirect respondents (e.g., other household members about whom primary respondents are asked), and do researchers need to provide the results or benefits of research to these indirect participants? At the same time, ethical issues raised by new technologies, such as geographic information systems (GIS), are affecting researchers undertaking any study, but are of special concern to longitudinal studies where geographical areas are more easily identifiable. Two discussions at the workshop—on incorporating biomedical testing and GIS into social research in developing countries—highlight some of the ethical dilemmas (see Box 2).

STRENGTHENING LONGITUDINAL EFFORTS

Because many longitudinal research efforts tend to be resource intensive and difficult, maximizing the returns to these efforts is a worthy aim. Much of the discussion at the workshop centered on eight ways in which longitudinal efforts could be strengthened: (1) building a strong, but flexible base survey; (2) increasing variables and types of data; (3) networking and collaborating; (4) linking data within and across studies; (5) strengthening research capacity; (6) expanding access through data sharing; (7) increasing data access and use through computer science innovations and technology; and (8) strengthening longitudinal research through funding mechanisms.

Building a Strong, but Flexible Base Survey

Many important findings that have emerged from longitudinal research were unintended at the onset of the study.[7] Because longitudinal studies involve multiple waves of data collection, researchers are able to incorporate changes in study communities during the observation period or employ technological developments to investigate a topic. Flexibility and adaptability are features of longitudinal research. The power of longitudinal data lies not just in repeated measures of the same variables, but also in the ability to add a rich set of non-time-varying covariates for analysis in new domains as well as contextual information for prespecified hypotheses. However, the ability to add on to a study or use data in ways originally unintended requires a strong research design—one that includes a broad range of carefully defined variables providing a solid base on which to build.

Strong study designs are central to researchers' ability to capitalize on opportunities that arise during the research process. Speaking of longitudinal studies in the United States, Willis argued the most successful studies have clear objectives and a solid base of information, with designs flexible enough to capitalize on any new opportunities accompanying theoretical and empirical developments or a changing context. A well-conceived core of variables increases the likelihood that additional research topics can be easily built in with additional questions or research modules and that collected waves of data can serve as baseline information for new programs, policies, or changes in the study environment.

Recent examples demonstrate the importance of building on a solid foundation. Even though economic shocks were not anticipated at the outset of the studies, researchers were able to, because of a strong foundation, examine carefully the economic crisis in Indonesia through RAND's Indonesian Family Life Survey (Frankenberg et al., 1998, 1999), and the increasing long-term poverty and need for changes in the social safety net in Russia through the Russian Longitudinal Monitoring Survey conducted by the University at North Carolina at Chapel Hill (Lokshin and Popkin, 1999; Popkin and Mroz, 1995). Likewise, in Mozambique researchers were able to detect the doubling of infant mortality in the study region during 2000, possibly related to the stress of the January and February floods,

---

[7]This section is based on presentations by Robert Willis, Monica Das Gupta, and Agnes Quisumbing.

BOX 2
Ethical Issues Associated with Adding Geocoding and Biomarkers to Longitudinal Research

The ethical issues raised by new technologies are affecting all kinds of research, but especially longitudinal studies where geographical areas are more easily identifiable. These issues described here are exacerbated by, but not unique to, longitudinal studies.

Geocoding and GIS data

Because of technological advances in the collection and use of geospatial data and the availability of geographic identifiers, researchers are increasingly incorporating geospatial data into survey data.* Not only are geospatial variables useful as analytical variables, but they also enhance research in two ways: by facilitating the linkage of independent datasets through common geospatial references (e.g., latitude-longitude coordinates, administrative area codes, or enumeration district codes) and by providing the basic information needed to generate other variables (such as those related to distance, availability, direction, and proximity of facilities).

The use of these techniques, however, raises two ethical considerations. First, it is more likely that study respondents could be identified through attributes, locations, or other information obtainable through these codes. And, second, it is more likely that data could be used for purposes other than those intended by the original data collectors, raising issues about informed consent.

Collecting Biomarkers

Scientific developments over the past few decades have dramatically increased researchers' abilities to collect biological data from testing of respondents requiring small amounts of biological material (such as blood spots and saliva).** These developments have not only helped researchers to provide better diagnoses of some infections and diseases than those based on self-reports or

---

*This section is based on the presentation by Stephen Matthews.

other measures, but also enabled them to examine some individual characteristics through simple biomarkers. The use of bioindicators in longitudinal social science and public health research raises the following questions:

- How much time elapses between taking the sample and getting the results? What are the implications of this timing for researchers? Do the results influence the timing of the next visit?
- How should researchers deal with inaccurate tests (such as false positive and false negatives)? Should tests be repeated? When? Under what conditions?
- Are the results of use to the individual respondent? Should respondents be given all results?
- What is the public health significance of the results? How does this affect researchers' obligations to individual participants?
- Do the results have social implications (e.g., social stigma) for respondents?
- Is treatment available or not? What does treatment require?
- Can researchers store blood or other samples for tests that are developed in the future? Are researchers obligated to store blood or other biological samples? For how long?
- Do researchers have to track respondents over time to provide them with results discovered later (either unanticipated ones or those that take time to show up)? For how long?
- Do researchers have an obligation to inform participants about very complex interactions between biological and social characteristics? What are the responsibilities of researchers when treatment for a particular condition requires both medical and social responses?
- What are researchers' obligations to secondary respondents or families that may be implicated in findings (such as those indicating the presence of HIV or susceptibility to hereditary diseases)?

**Based on presentations by Noreen Goldman and Stan Becker.

through the Manhica longitudinal community study in Mozambique (described in the presentation by Stephen Tollman).

The next step to strengthening longitudinal efforts involves developing research designs that not only accommodate serendipity, but also *encourage* it. Monica Das Gupta argued that the number of unintended findings with great consequence to knowledge and public well-being (Aaby, 1997) suggest that researchers should strive to develop designs that foster serendipity and unanticipated findings in the research process.

Increasing Variables and Types of Data

The addition of more or different variables to longitudinal data collection can increase the potential and use of longitudinal data. This is especially true when the added variables substantially improve researchers' ability to incorporate more accurate measures of important factors or test more complex models. Two specific examples of such variables were discussed at the workshop: geocoding and collecting biomarkers, particularly in conjunction with social surveys.

Stephen Matthews described how the use of geospatial data (data that indicates the physical location and characteristics of a community or site) strengthens longitudinal research by enabling researchers to create new variables and better measures, and to better model complex relationships. The heightened awareness of geospatial and geocoded data, the increasing availability of this data, and technologies to access and use it offer researchers opportunities to add value to existing data. Matthews argued that, when used properly, geospatial data enhances demographic modeling by incorporating geographic relationships and structure into analyses and improving the robustness and validity of spatial demographic modeling and longitudinal methods.

Matthews cautioned, however, that GIS is not a panacea. Selecting appropriate units of analysis and properly aggregating data to new units, accessing and integrating data, dealing with small sample sizes and data clusters, and recognizing problems in geospatial data (e.g., misspecified data, missing data, inconsistent geocodes) require theoretical and practical considerations. From a modeling perspective, GIS adds a huge overlay of complexity in terms of both spatial aggregation and identification.

Likewise, collecting bioindicators (such as blood or saliva samples), particularly in conjunction with social data greatly enhances the quality of several health measures and expands the range of research questions that can be addressed by researchers. Reporting on their experience of adding biomarker data to a broad longitudinal survey in Taiwan, Noreen Goldman and Maxine Weinstein described how they were able to address several limitations of social data, permitting them to incorporate individuals' health trajectories into their models; examine the relationships between social, economic, psychosocial, and physiological factors; and obtain markers across different physiological systems with recent information, using a large, nonclinical sample. Their experience collecting biomarkers in Taiwan was successful (acceptable response rates, high compliance with protocol, very few complaints from respondents) and promising for social and health research.

In short, achievement of study value will depend on additional variables contributing to, not detracting from, the major research goals, and the benefits of including such variables should outweigh the additional resources they entail.

Networking and Collaborating

The research potential of longitudinal data is greater when combining studies of different types or covering different topical or regional areas. By networking and collaborating across sites and study approaches, researchers can easily leverage longitudinal data, increasing their value. Networking of researchers involved in various studies facilitates the development of comparable datasets across study sites. The value of the research programs such as the (largely cross-sectional) World Fertility Surveys, Demographic and Health Surveys, and the World Bank's Living Standards Measurement Surveys has been enhanced by obtaining comparable data across countries, enabling comparative research. Perhaps with this advantage in mind, networks are emerging around various longitudinal studies.

The example of the INDEPTH network highlights the added value accrued through relationships between researchers at various sites or involved in projects in different types of data collection or objectives. Founded in November of 1998, INDEPTH is a network of longitudinal community field sites based on health and demographic surveillance systems to capitalize on the research and policy-informing capabilities organized by researchers from various field sites. The network not only provides an opportunity for sites to work with and learn from the experiences of other sites, but also promotes activities and technologies that enable researchers to exploit the comparative capabilities of the research. For example, the network has initiated a monograph series that adds value to findings from individual sites by presenting information (e.g., age-specific mortality rates and life tables) in a comparative manner, enabling researchers to identify seven distinct patterns of mortality in Africa (INDEPTH Network, 2002). INDEPTH plans to produce other volumes presenting demographic and health topics in a similar fashion. The topics include cause-specific mortality and a new initiative on malaria transmission intensity and the mortality burden in Africa, health equity, and migration patterns. These efforts can strengthen individual sites as well as promote standardized datasets and increase the potential for further cross-site comparisons and multisite research.

Recognizing the limitations of longitudinal community studies (primarily in terms of their limited geographical coverage), INDEPTH also is collaborating with the African Census Analysis Project[8] to capitalize on the opportunities for examining African populations by means of combining detailed longitudinal data from longitudinal community sites with the coverage of censuses. A collaborative effort between these two organizatons, which may focus on HIV/AIDS, is in the early stages.

Collaboration, which often builds on networks, occurs when one or more groups of researchers, using comparable datasets, carry out research in common or in conjunction with other groups. Plans are under way to initiate studies comparable to HRS/AHEAD in several European countries, expanding the uses of these data. Similar collaborations could be encouraged in developing countries.

Linking Data Within or Across Studies

Linking data to other sources of data in a study or in a particular site (such as data from another study, GIS or community level data) can add value by increasing, without additional data collection, the information available on individuals or other study units when common variables exist. Linking occurs within and across datasets.

Within a single dataset, researchers can link information on couples,

---

[8]The African Census Analysis Project (ACAP) is a joint initiative of the University of Pennsylvania and several African demographic research and training institutions. The main objective of this initiative is to consolidate African censuses to make them more accessible and increase their comparative potential.

family members, or households to increase research potential. Allan Hill argued that most analyses of longitudinal data fall short of exploiting their full potential by failing to build on linkages and other internal features of longitudinal designs. By linking and comparing couples' responses on desired and (subsequent) actual fertility in the Farafenni (Gambia) longitudinal community study, Hill demonstrated that discordant reporting of live births between men and women was significantly related to the woman's age and the time since the marriage, controlling for the man's age.[9] He illustrated how linking couples improved data quality (particularly age reporting of children), identified incomplete responses, and provided insight into complex family processes, such as polygyny and fostering, which vary over time. Although linking couples generated additional technical, theoretical, and ethical challenges for researchers, it added considerable value to existing studies.

In the study by Menken and her colleagues described earlier, linking data from two studies at the same site—one with detailed information on health and socioeconomic variables at one point in time and one with detailed information on mortality—enabled researchers to contribute to substantive (the influence of early characteristics on later survival probabilities) and methodological (the influence of the length of observation on findings) knowledge.

Particularly relevant to issues around linking data is the development of technologies for generating or handling data. The generation of common variables in multiple datasets through geocoding has already been discussed. Developments to ease the extensive technological demands of large and complex datasets, such as linked data, are presented in the later section "Increasing Data Access and Use Through Computer Science Innovations and Technology."

Strengthening Research Capacity

Efforts to expand the participation of developing country scientists in research and strengthen their analytical skills improves the quality of current research and research capacity in developing regions.

---

[9]The older the woman and the more time since marriage, the greater the predicted probability of discordant reporting, and the greater the predicted probability that the man will report more live births than the woman will.

As a first step, Francis Dodoo reminded workshop participants that capacity strengthening demands a conscientious effort by researchers to identify what communities and developing country scientists want. It is critical that researchers carefully define what capacity strengthening involves, what skills will be enhanced, and how these skills will be developed.

For example, Dodoo argued that capacity strengthening may require both training researchers to be sophisticated users of the technology required to manipulate and analyze data and training them to raise thoughtful and provocative research questions and to develop their own projects. These goals are different and require different strategies. The first involves technological and statistical skills; the second requires analytical and writing skills.

Studies differ in the strategies they employ to strengthen research capacity. Most current longitudinal community studies explicitly incorporate local research development into their projects; indeed, strengthening local research capacity is often a key objective guiding these studies (as discussed earlier in the section "Relationships with Communities and Respondents"). Researchers carrying out panel and cohort studies have generally worked with research institutions in developing countries rather than individual scientists. All studies require that researchers and funding agencies grapple with issues of project ownership and ensure that developing country collaborators receive due credit for their work on joint projects.[10]

A serious commitment to capacity strengthening requires integrating these goals into the criteria, review process, and evaluation of research and supporting grants. The following two examples of supportive strategies for capacity building presented at the workshop demonstrate the explicit plans and commitment required to strengthen capacity successfully.

First, Kenneth Bridbord described the strategy for improving the research capacity of scientists from developing nations at the U.S. National Institute of Health's Fogarty International Center (FIC). Serving the overall goal of "promot[ing] and support[ing] scientific research and training internationally to reduce disparities in global health," the FIC promotes training of scientists and health professionals through training and research grants, international training grants for U.S. citizens, and institutional grants to universities and nonprofit research institutions with demonstrated

---

[10]This paragraph is based on the presentation of Francis Dodoo.

collaboration with foreign research institutions. The program is built on five principles for capacity building in developing country scientists:

1. a long-term effort and commitment
2. in-country coordination with local and community leadership
3. promotion of "South to South" collaboration
4. training, networking, and mentoring
5. support for a wide range of health professionals (including nurses, nurse midwives, laboratory staff, counselors, physicians, traditional healers, program administrators).

Second, Cheikh Mbacke argued that, "because they entail long-term involvement with communities in geographically defined areas, longitudinal studies have great potential for building both individual and institutional capacity." Speaking specifically about longitudinal community studies in Africa, he highlighted the need for explicit strategies for capacity strengthening in order to exploit the opportunities for capacity development inherent in these projects. He then presented six critical aspects of capacity building at African longitudinal sites.

The two most important requirements of capacity building are a solid institutional grounding and a capacity for effectively mobilizing resources. The second two most important requirements are demonstrating the relevance and benefit of the research to the local community and reducing the costs of research endeavors through innovative data collection, changes in methodology, and new technologies. The last two important aspects of capacity building are attracting and keeping scientists, especially local scientists, and enhancing networking capacities to increase the analytic potential of the data and project (for example, through comparative studies) and to promote growth opportunities.

Expanding Access Through Data Sharing

Data sharing, or making data available to secondary users, has substantial potential for quickly advancing longitudinal efforts and the related scientific and policy benefits. However, data sharing also raises several concerns about protecting respondents and ensuring data quality. A critical question addressed at the workshop was: how do researchers balance the tension between protecting the property rights of producers of the data and serving the desires of secondary users, including the public, to get the maximum use and benefit out of the data?

Christine Bachrach identified some of the benefits and costs associated with data sharing. Six benefits of data sharing were discussed, specifically how data sharing:

1. advances science
2. promotes timely analysis and dissemination of data
3. increases the speed with which results get out
4. facilitates linking independent datasets
5. increases efficient use of scarce resources
6. promotes hands-on training opportunities.

The costs, or drawbacks, of data sharing include four issues:

1. Data sharing can pose a threat to the perceived intellectual property rights of investigators.
2. Data sharing reduces the control of the principal investigator and the scientific community over the use of data, increasing the possibility for misuse, misleading results, or bad research based on the data.
3. The process of preparing, documenting, disseminating, and supporting data incurs monetary costs.
4. Data sharing can pose potential risks to privacy of research participants.

The issues raised in this list highlight a core issue in data sharing: successful data sharing requires balancing the potentially competing interests of three interest groups—the data controllers (collectors and primary users), the data users, and the data subjects (or respondent community). In his presentation, Kobus Herbst outlined the different interests and roles of these three groups (see Figure 1).

Data controllers, those who collect and maintain the data, are obliged to produce high-quality data, invest in the local community, attract and keep quality researchers, and protect respondents. These obligations and the nontrivial investments that data controllers make give them the right to use the data before others have access to it. Allowing some time for collectors to work with the data is important for ensuring the quality of the data, incorporating measures to protect the security of respondents, and developing the necessary codebooks and instructions for using the data.

Data Collectors
- Producing high-quality data
- Generating useful scientific findings (advancing science and policy)
- Attracting and keeping good researchers and staff
- Protecting respondents
- Sustaining the project

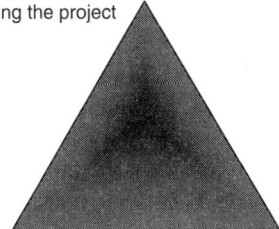

Data Users
- Advancing science
- Setting research-based policies
- Examining aspects of data not being looked at by others

Data Subjects
- Enjoying confidentiality
- Being fully informed about the uses of the information provided (informed consent)
- Seeing benefits of research (improved health and well-being)
- Avoiding harm

FIGURE 1 Interests of data collectors, data users and data subjects in longitudinal research projects.
SOURCE: Based on presentation by Kobus Herbst.

Data users, including secondary users, policy makers, and the general public, are interested in recognizing the benefits of data as quickly as possible. Broad use of data reinforces scientific inquiry, a diversity of perspectives of approaches, and investigations other than those planned by the data collectors. Data sharing serves the interests of this group by increasing the knowledge base in a timely manner.

The interests of data subjects include both ethical dimensions and the rights to information. Confidentiality, privacy, and safety are key concerns of data subjects and their communities. Data sharing can compromise the ability of data collectors to ensure these protections. Yet, respondents also have an interest in receiving the benefits of the research—which is encouraged and expedited through data sharing.

These issues again highlight the distinctions between cohort and panel studies, on the one hand, and longitudinal community studies, on the other. Whereas cohort and panel studies in developing countries tend to be fairly accessible to secondary and public users within a few years of data collection, longitudinal community studies have remained under the tight grip of the researchers and institutions collecting the data. These different data-sharing practices arise largely from the different features of these studies. As discussed in previous sections, longitudinal community studies often work with massive amounts of data that are continually collected, and they have goals and relationships with communities that differ greatly from those associated with other longitudinal studies thus data collectors involved with those studies face multiple demands. Again, because they are located in small physical areas, researchers working with longitudinal community studies face added challenges in protecting their respondents.

Many workshop participants agreed that the dilemma of competing interests can be resolved by adopting explicit strategies and creative models that reflect the various needs and concerns and that are appropriate for the topics and goals of studies. Workshop participants then discussed the various approaches to data sharing now in use (generally from most accessible to most restrictive):

- Datasets are available on the Internet.
- Data can be acquired through a formal request process (with or without a charge).
- Variables that could be used to identify respondents (ID variables) or communities (such as geocodes) can be removed.
- Data can be made available to secondary users who come to multipurpose data centers or enclaves.
- Subsets of data in the form of specific modules or variables can be made available
- Data at various levels of aggregation can be made available.
- Users can request summary tables or specific analyses that are then provided by data custodians.

Thus, depending on the research interests and critical issues associated with a particular dataset or study, different strategies of data sharing can be developed to promote wider use of data without compromising the confidentiality of respondents, the property rights of primary users, or the quality of research. To date, removing identifying variables from shared data, especially public access samples, is the most common approach.

Data collectors also have responsibilities for facilitating use of their data. The Demographic and Health Surveys are currently available on the

Internet to any interested users that complete a short form. Martin Vaessen described issues that the DHS has addressed in making these data widely available. Specfiically, Vaessen pointed out that data should be provided in usable formats, and multiple formats when possible, to be most useful. Users also need the tools required to use the data, including software, training, and documentation. The documentation should address information about the contents and general features of the data, the history of its collection and use, and its nuances.

Determining when data should be made available is a critical consideration that requires a compromise between the various interests just described. Having a clearly set schedule that details when data will be more broadly available and the procedures for accessing them is perhaps the most important consideration.

Several workshop participants mentioned that often data-sharing practices are determined by the funding agencies of a project; expectations about when the data will enter the public domain is included in the original agreement. Christine Bachrach suggested that funding agencies become more involved with creative models to encourage data sharing and that they work data-sharing expectations into the granting process (as is currently the case with many panel studies supported by the U.S. National Institutes of Health).

Increasing Data Access and Use Through Computer Science Innovations and Technology

Many issues of data sharing, particularly the tension between primary and secondary users, can be addressed through improved technologies for collecting, maintaining and using longitudinal data.[11] Although these issues are not specific to longitudinal data, in view of the amount of data produced in longitudinal studies, the technology and processes for managing and analyzing data are particularly salient. Once the intensive data collection and management requirements are reduced, data collectors can spend more time analyzing data. Many longitudinal community sites and the INDEPTH network are currently developing mechanisms for more efficient data storage and management. As primary users shift their emphasis from data handling to analysis with better data management and

---

[11]This section is based on presentations by Bruce MacLeod and Sam Clark.

analysis software, their returns increase and the prospects of data sharing are enhanced.

Reducing the time and costs associated with data storage and retrieval is critical for the long-term success of longitudinal community sites. Bruce MacLeod calculated that data storage and retrieval currently account for 10-40 percent of research budgets. These figures are likely to go up if biomarkers or extra security measures are included.

Currently, software to automate construction of data management systems building on consistency logic and basic data types is being developed in the field by experienced users. Simplifying data management of single sites is an important goal for software design; however, a main objective is to develop templates and other mechanisms that facilitate standardized data formats (particularly definitions of key variables and data storage logic) across studies, thereby supporting cross-country comparisons and linkages between datasets.

A basic building block of this project is a relational data model, described by Sam Clark, with the capacity for self-generation (and change) of relational variables with minimal syntax. The Structural Population Event History Register (SPEHR) is an example.[12] Requests for summary tables or specific analyses are filled by data custodians. Workshop participants discussed seven design considerations for relational data model for longitudinal population data:

- standards and comparability: compatible data definitions and storage structures across datasets
- flexibility and extensibility: ability to manage data with a wide range of realities around time dimension, structure dimension (marriages, households, residences), and relationships
- self-documentation: management system that automatically generates descriptions of data, logic, and metadata.

---

[12] The SPEHR is a relational data model being developed by Sam Clark and his colleagues. The model is built on several components: events (birth, death), multievent processes, item-episodes (residency at place X from time 1 to time 2, marital union from date of union to separation), experiences (the manner in which an item-episode is affected by an event or vice versa), shared experiences, and attributes that change over time. A working demonstration is available at http://www.samclark.net/SPEHR/SPEHR.htm.

- easy maintenance: automated day-to-day maintenance tasks that include adding, editing, and deleting data and data structures; verifying data integrity; and generating operational reports
- security: system that includes partitioning of data into secured units and legally inaccessible units and centralized control over data
- validity: no duplication of data and checks for validity
- analysis-friendly: user-friendly software based on intuitive design, easily recognizable views of the data, and defined summary measures and analytical building blocks, and defined output data formats

The ultimate goal of relational models and supportive software is to facilitate the sharing and comparing of data from different populations to improve the scientific and research base on demographic and health issues.

Strengthening Longitudinal Research Through Funding Mechanisms

A recurrent and important theme emerged throughout the discussions of each topic covered in this section of the report. For each topic, workshop participants recognized the importance of support from funding agencies to fully realize the objectives identified. If sustainability, capacity building, data sharing, community involvement, linking, and networking are worthy goals, funding agencies should encourage and support them through more precise and explicit strategies in proposals and award criteria. For example, sustainability strategies, including a fixed time limit for funding and a plan to shift to local funding mechanisms, should be built into original proposals to encourage in-country support and less reliance on international funding agencies. If capacity strengthening is a priority, plans for strengthening capacity, including a clear definition of what it entails, should be explicit in the proposals, funding criteria, and evaluations of the project. The same is true for the goals of networking and data sharing, dissemination of results back to the community, and collaborative work. Not only will these strategies enable researchers and funding agencies to better realize their own objectives, but incorporating aspects of interest into the funding mechanisms will help researchers determine which longitudinal approaches are most appropriate given the set of objectives on the table.

CONCLUSION

The main goal of this workshop was to compare the strengths and weaknesses of different longitudinal approaches—specifically, panel, cohort, and longitudinal community studies. These approaches differ in their objectives for research and community participation, the study populations and samples, the potential for addressing various research questions, and the ethical concerns with which researchers must grapple. This report has highlighted how these approaches compare in confronting several challenges faced by longitudinal researchers and in adding value to existing and future longitudinal efforts. A clear theme of the workshop was the importance of using longitudinal approaches that best fit the research questions being asked or the overall goals of the project, which may include aspects of community strengthening and local investment along with the scientific objectives.

A second major theme that emerged was the importance of multiple research approaches to enhance scientific progress and improve the well-being of individuals through effective policies. Workshop participants identified how the weaknesses in one approach could be easily offset by linking the data collected using that approach with other data collected using similar or different approaches. Issues of access to data—clearly a critical need in increasing the use (and value) of longitudinal data—resurfaced throughout the workshop as an area that needs more careful and critical attention, particularly as it affects the ability to protect the confidentiality of respondents and communities. Overall, the workshop emphasized the importance of careful designs that provide the best science and information while protecting respondents and the communities in which they live, whatever the approach.

REFERENCES

Aaby, P.
    1997   Bandim: An unplanned longitudinal study. Pp. 276-296 in *Prospective Community Studies in Developing Countries*, M. Das Gupta, P. Aaby, M. Garenne, and G. Pison. Oxford: Clarendon Press.
Adair, L.S., C.W. Kuwaza, and J. Borja.
    2001   Maternal energy stores and diet composition during pregnancy program adolescent blood pressure. *Circulation* 104:1034-1039.
Adair, L.S., and D.K. Guilkey
    1997   Age-specific determinants of stunting in Filipino children. *Journal of Nutrition* 127:314-320.
Alderman, H., J.R. Berhman, H.-P. Kohler, J.A. Maluccio, and S.C. Watkins
    2001   Attrition in longitudinal household survey data. *Demographic Research* 5(4):80-124.

Aziz, K.M.A., and W.H. Mosley
    1997 The history, methodology, and main findings of the Matlab project in Bangladesh. Pp. 28-53 in *Prospective Community Studies in Developing Countries*, M. Das Gupta, P. Aaby, M. Garenne, and G. Pison, eds. Oxford: Clarendon Press.

Barker, D.J.P.
    1998 In utero programming of chronic disease. *Clinical Science* 95:115-28.

Bell, C., K. Ge, and B.M. Popkin.
    2001 Weight gain and its predictors in Chinese adults. *International Journal of Obesity* 25:1079-1086.

Cantrelle, P.
    1969 Étude démographique dans la région du Sine-Saloum (Sénégal). État-civil et observations démographiques. *Travaux et Documents de L'ORSTOM*, No. 1. Paris: ORSTOM.

Das Gupta, M., P. Aaby, M. Garenne, and G. Pison
    1997 *Prospective Community Studies in Developing Countries.* Oxford: Clarendon Press.

Frankenberg, E., K. Beegle, B. Sikoki, and D. Thomas
    1998 *Health, Family Planning and Well-Being in Indonesia during an Economic Crisis: Early Results from the Indonesian Family Life Survey.* DRU-2013-FGI/NICHD/UNFPA. Santa Monica, CA: RAND.

Frankenberg, E., D. Thomas, and K. Beegle
    1999 *The Real Costs of Indonesia's Economic Crisis: Preliminary Findings From the Indonesian Family Life Survey.* DRU-2064-NIA/NICHD. Santa Monica, CA: RAND.

Garenne, M., and P. Cantrelle
    1997 Three decades of reseach on population and health: The ORSTOM experience in rural Senegal, 1962-1991. Pp. 235-252 in *Prospective Community Studies in Developing Countries*, M. Das Gupta, P. Aaby, M. Garenne, and G. Pison, eds. Oxford: Clarendon Press.
    2001 Prospective studies of communities: Their unique potential for studying the health transition: Reflections from the ORSTOM experience in Senegal. Pp. 251-285 in *The Health Transition: Methods and Measures, Proceedings of an International Workshop*, J. Cleland and A.G. Hill, eds. London.

Garenne, M., and E. Koumans
    1997 Appendix: Prospective community studies in developing countries: A survey of surveys. Pp. 297-338 in *Prospective Community Studies in Developing Countries*, M. Das Gupta, P. Aaby, M. Garenne, and G. Pison, eds. Oxford: Clarendon Press.

Guo, X., T.A. Mroz, B.M. Popkin, and F. Zhai
    2000 Structural changes in the impact of income on food consumption in China, 1989-93. *Economic Development and Cultural Change* 48:737-760.

INDEPTH Network
    2002 *Population and Health in Developing Countries, Volume 1: Population, Health, and Survival in INDEPTH Sites.* Ottawa: International Development Research Centre.

Kahn, K., and S. Tollman
  1998 The INDEPTH Network: A Comparative Perspective on Field Sites in Africa, Asia, Latin America, and the Middle East. Unpublished manuscript.
Lokshin, M., and B.M. Popkin
  1999 The emerging underclass in the Russian Federation: Income dynamics 1992-1996. *Economic Development and Cultural Change* 47:803-829.
Lokshin, M., K.M. Harris, and B.M. Popkin
  2000 Single mothers in Russia: Household strategies for coping with poverty. *World Development* 28:2183-2198.
Martorell, R.
  1995 Results and implications of the INCAP follow-up study. *Journal of Nutrition* 125(4 Suppl):1127S-1138S.
Martorell, R., J.P. Habicht, and J.A. Rivera
  1995 History and design of the INCAP longitudinal study (1969-77) and its follow-up (1988-89). *Journal of Nutrition* 125(4 Suppl):1027S-1041S.
Martorell, R., J.A. Rivera, and C.K. Lutter
  1990 Interaction of diet and disease in child growth. Pp. 307-321 in *Breastfeeding, Nutrition, Infection and Infant Growth in Developed and Emerging Countries*. S.A. Atkinson, L.A. Hanson, and R.K. Chandra, eds. St John's, Newfoundland: ARTS Biomedical Publishers and Distributors.
Mendez, M.E., and L.S. Adair
  1999 Severity and timing of stunting in infancy and performance on IQ and school achievement tests in late childhood. *Journal of Nutrition* 129:1555-1562.
Mosley, W.H.
  1989 *Population Laboratories for Community Health Research*. Working paper number 51. Mexico City: Population Council.
Popkin, B., and T. Mroz
  1995 Poverty and the economic transition in the Russian Federation. *Economic Development and Cultural Change* 44:1-31.
Popkin, B.M., M.K. Richards, and C. Monteiro
  1996 Stunting is associated with overweight in children of four nations that are undergoing the nutrition transition. *Journal of Nutrition* 126:3009-3016.
Ramakrishnan, U., R. Martorell, D.G. Schroeder, and R. Flores
  1999a Roles of intergenerational effects on linear growth. *Journal of Nutrition* 129(2S Suppl):544S-549S.
Ramakrishnan, U., H. Barnhart, D.G. Schroeder, A.D. Stein, and R. Martorell
  1999b Early childhood nutrition, education and fertility milestones in Guatemala. *Journal of Nutrition* 129(11):2196-2202
Ruel, M.T., J.A. Rivera, J.P. Habicht, and R. Martorell
  1995 Differential response to early nutrition supplementation: Long-term effects on height at adolescence. International Journal of Epidemiology 24(2):404-412.
Schroeder, D.G., R. Martorell, and R. Flores
  1999 Infant and child growth and fatness and fat distribution in Guatemalan adults. *American Journal of Epidemiology* 149(2): 177-185.

Scrimshaw, N.S., and M.A. Guzman
    1997   A comparison of supplementary feeding and medical care of preschool children in Guatemala, 1959-1964. Pp. 133-156 in *Prospective Community Studies in Developing Countries*, M. Das Gupta, P. Aaby, M. Garenne, and G. Pison, eds. Oxford: Clarendon Press.

Taylor, C.E., and C. De Sweemer
    1997   Lessons from Narangwal about primary health care, family planning, and nutrition. Pp. 101-132 in *Prospective Community Studies in Developing Countries*, M. Das Gupta, P. Aaby, M. Garenne, and G. Pison, eds. Oxford: Clarendon Press.

Willis, R.J.
    1999   Theory confronts data: How the HRS is shaped by the economics of aging, and how the economics of aging will be shaped by the HRS. *Labour Economics* (special issue)6(2):119-145.

Wyon, J.B.
    1997   Determinants of rates of early childhood sickness and death, and of long birth intervals: Evidence from the Khanna study, rural Punjab, India, 1954-1969. Pp. 54-80 in *Prospective Community Studies in Developing Countries*, M. Das Gupta, P. Aaby, M. Garenne, and G. Pison, eds. Oxford: Clarendon Press.

Wyon, J.B., and J.E. Gordon
    1971   *The Khanna Study: Population Problems in the Rural Punjab*. Cambridge, MA: Harvard University Press.

PART II

PAPERS

Demographic Analysis of Community, Cohort, and Panel Data from Low-Income Countries: Methodological Issues

Andrew Foster
Department of Economics and Community Health
Brown University

In any examination of the methodological issues related to the use of longitudinal data, it is helpful to consider three distinct uses for these data: measurement, evaluation, and structural analysis. As discussed in greater detail later in this paper, measurement focuses on the description of patterns of demographic change; evaluation is concerned primarily with measuring the consequences of policies or programs; and structural analysis involves testing and measuring underlying mechanisms or structures. This grouping is somewhat arbitrary, and, arguably, most demographic analyses involve more than one of these purposes, but the categorization is useful, because it helps to clarify the extent to which different forms of demographic data are linked to their eventual use. In particular, dissimilarities in the appropriateness of different data collection strategies are highest in areas of measurement, more moderate for evaluation, and somewhat limited in the context of structural analysis. This approach also helps to highlight the essential role played by longitudinal data collection in general as a basis for undertaking structural analysis. Specifically, it is argued that longitudinal data are critical for the modeling and analysis of the temporal antecedents of current behaviors and that clarifying the nature of these temporal antecedents provides important leverage for disentangling the mechanisms underlying demographic behavior.

This paper examines three categories of longitudinal data collection: panel, cohort, and community studies. These forms of data collection are distinguished as a group because they follow respondents over time. They are distinguished from each other by the criterion used to include individuals in the sample.

Panel studies generally use a representative sample of households from a broad region or nation at a particular point in time. Household members are then tracked and reinterviewed over time, regardless, given logistical considerations, of whether they have moved or otherwise changed their living arrangements. Such studies tend to be large in size and general-purpose in nature.

A cohort study follows a similar procedure in tracking individuals but is directed toward a specific group of individuals such as those born or married at a particular point in time, although supplementary information on other people residing with the primary respondent also may be collected. These studies tend to focus initially on relatively specific research questions, but they sometimes broaden over time to become multipurpose in nature.

A community study, by contrast, interviews individuals or households in a particular location and tracks entries and exits into this population, but it undertakes limited, if any, follow-up of participants leaving the region. Like cohort studies, community surveys usually are designed with a fairly narrow purpose in mind, such as the design and testing of a particular set of interventions, but they can later evolve into or provide a basis for more general-purpose data collection activities.

MEASUREMENT

The role of longitudinal data in measurement, as noted, is one of describing patterns of demographic change. *Measurement*, as the term is used in this paper, includes the computation of vital rates and other aspects of individual and household welfare, the distribution of these measures both within and across populations, and, most critically for a discussion of longitudinal data, changes in these measures over time. Although measurement in this sense may be considered a kind of precursor or motivation for more detailed evaluative or structural analysis, it has important purposes in its own right in characterizing and comparing different societies and for purposes of planning.

Measurement is not often listed as one of the key benefits of longitudinal data collection, but for certain purposes longitudinal data are critical, such as to track mobility. For example, a recent study examined the distribution of welfare changes in India over the last 30 years using panel data from rural India (Foster and Rosenzweig, 2001a). A series of census and other surveys such as the National Sample Survey for India provide the opportunity to measure changes in the distribution of income over time. From these surveys, investigators may, for example, establish whether rural poverty rates in India are increasing or decreasing over time and whether poverty rates are declining differentially in areas with higher agricultural productivity growth. For attributes such as sex, cohort, or, to a lesser extent, schooling that are fixed over time, one also can examine whether members of the groups as a whole did relatively well or poorly over a given interval. Such data, however, can say little about the relative gains or losses of groups in society that are more fluid over time.

Longitudinal data seem critical in evaluating whether income in poor households, for example, has declined relative to income in better-off households. Retrospective data can be useful for examining mobility with respect to relatively salient and well-defined events such as place of residence. In some cases, retrospective data may be the only or the most cost-effective way to construct such measures. But retrospective data seem particularly problematic for the evaluation of differential income mobility, because it would be a significant challenge to obtain accurate retrospective reports of income and expenditures. Moreover, because of attrition and household division, it would be difficult to use retrospective data to establish appropriate weights for the purpose of obtaining population estimates of previous income or income growth over a previous interval. For example, the average 1970 household income of individuals in a representative sample of individuals in 1980 will tend to exceed the actual average 1970 household income to the extent that large households are more likely than small households to divide. With retrospective data on household division rates, one could in principle correct these estimates, but there would be no way of correcting for households whose members had all migrated or died in the intervening years.

The ability to capture changes over time in individual, household, or community attributes does not appear to be an important distinguishing characteristic of the three types of data collection considered here. But a key requirement in the use of longitudinal data for measurement is a clear delimitation of the population being measured, and it is evident that these three forms of longitudinal data collection capture mobility in very different sets of populations. Not only is this true in the sense that different groups of people are being followed over time using the three approaches, but also important differences arise in the extent to which data collected from the relevant sample may be used to draw appropriate inferences about larger populations.

The issue of representativeness is dealt with most cleanly in the context of national panel surveys, though the discussion here can be easily modified to refer to large-scale surveys at less than a national level (such as a rural panel). As long as sufficient care is taken in drawing an appropriately representative sample in the first place, appropriately weighted rates of mobility, for example, starting from the initial period for a panel, are representative of population mobility.

Even in this case, however, important caveats must be addressed. The first is well understood: the quality of measurement of transitions over time will depend on the investigator's ability to follow individuals over time. Fortunately, recent experience from several panel surveys has provided substantial insight into the causes and consequences of attrition in panel surveys. The experience of the Indonesian Family Life Survey (IFLS) is particularly well documented (Thomas et al., 2002). This survey provides ample evidence that attrition is nonrandom for key observables in the baseline survey and that departure from the sample region, a key cause of attrition, is nonrandom for subsequent outcomes. In particular, as might be anticipated, the people who are lost to migration tend to have extreme outcomes—that is, substantially better or worse outcomes than for those who stay. The costs of following study participants who have left their hometown but not the country is high but not prohibitive, amounting to about a 20 percent increase in cost per interview in the context of the IFLS.

The second issue, which is more problematic, lies in the need to augment a panel survey so that it remains representative over time. For example, in a panel survey conducted in 1980, 1990, and 2000, population-level estimates of mobility between 1980 and 1990 and between 1980 and 2000 may be constructed using the 1980 sample weights. However, unless the 1990 panel is itself representative of the relevant population, inferences from this panel about mobility between 1990 and 2000 may be inappropriate. For some purposes, it may be possible to fix this problem by appropriately adjusting the sample weights, but for units of analysis such as the village in settings in which in-migration is common, it is necessary to include a sample of in-migrant households whose 1990-2000 mobility would not otherwise be captured. Even when an appropriate weighting system is available, the fact that the weights applied to particular households are likely to vary increasingly over time implies that population estimates tend to become increasingly variable and particularly sensitive to the presence of outliers.

Third, analysis of panel data is especially complex when considering changes over time in measures that are most naturally aggregated to the level of the household. For example, how does one measure income change in subsistence economies or other settings in which individual wage or salary data are unlikely to be available? If a landed agricultural household divides, the corresponding subhouseholds that started as a single unit with a single income measure may end up with very different levels of income in a subsequent round. Under these circumstances, estimates of income mobility at the individual, household, or dynastic (i.e., by adding together the incomes of the split-off households) levels may be quite different.

Finally, for some purposes it may be useful to construct a panel based on physical rather than social households. Such an approach would have some procedural advantages in that points in space are by definition immobile and therefore problems of attrition do not typically arise (although changes in topography such as the movement of the river may make a particular location inherently uninteresting for most purposes). This approach has been recommended by the World Bank as a desirable sampling scheme in developing countries (Glewwe and Grosh, 2000). However, whether this is indeed sensible depends on the questions to be answered. It seems a reasonable approach for asking questions about transitions that are spatially defined—such as whether relatively poor or isolated villages grow more or less rapidly on average over a particular interval. However, if an investigator is fundamentally interested in measuring the transitions faced by individuals, which seems reasonable in the context of most demographic analysis, then sampling social households and tracking individuals seems critical.

Many of these panel data issues apply in some degree to measurement in the context of community datasets and cohort studies. However, there are key differences between panel data and these other forms of longitudinal data collection in the extent to which they are generalizable to large populations. A cohort study can, of course, be representative of a group of people born at a particular point in time (or married at a particular point in time if that is the basis on which the cohort is drawn), but its findings cannot be easily generalized to the experience of other cohorts. Depending on the relative importance of changes that are common to cohorts (such as the process of aging) versus changes that are time-dependent and thus affect cohorts at different ages, the experience of one cohort may or may not be similar to those of other neighboring cohorts. Other, more subtle aspects of generalizability exist as well. To return to income mobility, average income growth in households of a particular cohort need not be representative of income mobility in the population as a whole at a particular point in time, because households with one member born in a particular year do not constitute a randomly selected sample of households.

Similarly, a community-level survey will be representative of the experience of a particular community at a particular point in time and can be used to establish changes in that community over time. But the experience of one community is not necessarily representative of other communities, and anyone using data from a single community has no obvious way of obtaining statistical measures of the extent of cross-community variability and thus of how different a particular community is likely to be from some average community in the relevant region. Compared with panel and cohort surveys, community surveys also have particular disadvantages in their treatment of out-migrants. Any measure of income mobility for individuals or communities, for example, will be problematic, because a community survey does not measure the experience of individuals and households who leave the community. In practice, one would expect the mobility experience of these individuals to be quite different from those who stay.

Measurement on a limited geographic scale also may have disadvantages from the perspective of measurement on a repeated cross-sectional basis given mobility. The idea is that even if one does not follow out-migrants from a national panel survey, a reasonable sample of both the sending and receiving areas is achieved. Thus, as long as the panel is augmented with a new sample to be representative at, say, the village level, it will capture on average the experience of out-migrants from the original sample areas. The panel component for these individuals is lost (because the in-migrants to sample villages will not be linked with out-migrants from other sample villages), but this is not a problem from the perspective of measurement on a repeated cross-sectional basis. The more limited the geographic area being considered, the more likely one is to lose even this type of information on mobile members of society.

But nonrepresentativeness need not imply that community surveys are unimportant for purposes of measurement. The frequency with which data from the Matlab study area in rural Bangladesh are used to characterize and validate overall changes in demographic rates in Bangladesh (see, for example, Cleland et al., 1994) suggests that such surveys play an important role in measurement. One of several reasons for this role is that survey costs in a contiguous geographic area are clearly lower than those in a nationally representative sample. Second, a study's investment in fixed resources within a particular community and long-run employment for workers may be more feasible in a community survey, possibly increasing the quality of workers who can be retained as well as the incentives to maintain quality. Long-term employment of survey workers also may increase data quality by increasing trust between survey workers and respondents. Third, the presence of an accurate census and persistent infrastructural support in a particular region at a particular point in time provides a useful basis for complementary analyses such as the development of specific-purpose longitudinal studies or qualitative analysis. Clearly, then, community surveys have had and will continue to have a critical role to play in measurement in developing countries without adequate censuses and vital registration systems.

EVALUATION

The second category of longitudinal data analysis—evaluation—provides the most commonly cited rationale for the collection of such data. At the heart of this rationale is the practical need to obtain, for policy design, estimates of program effects, coupled with the recognition that policies and programs are, in the absence of carefully designed intervention studies, likely to be systematically placed. This likelihood is known in the economics literature as the problem of endogenous program placement and incorporates deliberate attempts to target particular programs to particular areas (such as placing family planning clinics in high-fertility areas—see Gertler and Molyneaux, 1994), the tendency of people to live in places providing services they are likely to use (Rosenzweig and Wolpin, 1988), and correlations between outcome measures and programmatic variables that arise indirectly from underlying community attributes such as accessibility by road. Central to this approach is the notion that measurement of the effect is more important than understanding the underlying mechanisms responsible for the effect.

A short methodological digression on the underlying approach provides a useful foundation for a discussion later in this paper of the relative merits of different sorts of data. The underlying principle of this work is that some basic outcome of interest that is measured at two points in time, y_{it}, is a roughly linear function of a series of attributes x_{it}, the presence or absence of a program p_{it}, and a residual capturing fixed μ_i and time variant ε_{it} unobservables influencing the outcome in question:

(1) $\quad y_{it} = \beta x x_{it} + \beta p p_{it} + \mu_i + \varepsilon_{it}$

The basic statistical problem is that the correlation between the program variable p_{it} and the unobservables implies that standard linear methods will yield a biased measure of the effect of the program. In the special case in which the allocation of the program is correlated with the underlying fixed effects, in which the program is introduced or modified over time, and in which the linearity assumption is plausible, program effects may be measured through a differencing procedure or by including dummy variables at the level of aggregation of the community. Alternatively, if there is reason to suspect that changes in the program between periods t and $t + 1$ are correlated with the initial time-varying component ε_{it}, it is possible to combine differencing with an instrumental variables procedure, using as instruments the initial values of the x_{it} variables.

A close look at the assumptions that must be made to apply this approach suggests that the principle of using over-time variation to evaluate program effects does not intrinsically require access to individual-level longitudinal data. To the extent that the program being evaluated is available to all members of a community, little may be gained from being able to follow study participants over time. A comparison of the fertility behavior of a given woman before and after the introduction of a family planning clinic is likely to be less informative about the effects of the family planning program than a comparison between women of similar ages at two points in time. Indeed, what appears to be the earliest application of this approach to the evaluation of demographic programs considered the effects of family planning expenditures on fertility at the level of the district in Taiwan (Schultz, 1973). Other work in this area has made effective use of repeated cross-sectional data aggregated to the level of the community (Pitt et al., 1993).

Because the underlying methodology effectively incorporates the assumption of a single, well-defined coefficient reflecting program impact, the issue of representativeness that plays a critical role in a comparison of different forms of longitudinal data collection for the purpose of measurement does not play a decisive role here. If program effects are importantly heterogeneous, then different types of longitudinal data will yield different measures of the effect. However, admitting that the effects may be importantly heterogeneous and that one cares about the magnitude of the effect rather than just, for example, its sign, raises a host of new difficulties. In particular, the process of differencing or the application of instrumental variables will yield a coefficient from a particular dataset that is not representative of the average effect of the program on the corresponding population. For example, the process of differencing over time to measure the effects of a family planning clinic effectively removes from the dataset all villages with family planning clinics in both the initial and final periods, and thus a program effect obtained from differencing village data yields at best an estimate of the program effect in those villages that experienced a change, not the average effect on all villages in the relevant population.

Although representativeness does not therefore helpfully distinguish the three forms of longitudinal data collection, significant differences can be found in the relative suitability of these approaches to the assumptions and data requirements of the proposed methods. For a panel survey, to the extent that the evaluation is of a community-level program, panel data may not be ideal for evaluating program effects; one needs instead a representative sample of the population at two points in time. Thus if there is sufficient migration or change in household composition, the panel data will not yield representative estimates unless investigators deliberately try to resample and apply the appropriate weights.

Cohort data present similar problems for the evaluation of community-level programs. But additional issues arise if program effects are likely to be significantly age-related. As noted, changes in fertility in a given cohort over time are likely to have much more to do with changes in age and the stock of children than with the introduction of a family planning program. At the very least, the linearity assumption embodied in equation (1) is likely to be violated in cohort data if a differencing approach is used to measure the impact of family planning programs on fertility. Yet cohort studies may be particularly well suited to stratified sampling designs in which treated individuals (i.e., those making use of the program) are relatively rare within a population. By ensuring that treated individuals are oversampled within a particular cohort, an investigator can maximize statistical power for a given sample size.

From this perspective, community-based longitudinal data collection seems ideal for purposes of evaluation. By deliberately tracking entrants, exits, and relevant behaviors in a particular community, researchers can address problems of shifting population and compare appropriate groups at different points in time. They are also able, in the context of a community-based survey, to deliberately design interventions, such as the Matlab family planning program in rural Bangladesh (see Menken and Phillips, 1990) and the nutrition supplement experiments in rural Guatemala (see Pollitt et al., 1995). Like for evaluation, a focus on a particular region enhances the opportunity to introduce complementary studies such as longitudinal surveys or qualitative work that may inform the evaluative process.

Set against these positive attributes is the relatively limited geographic coverage generally provided by community-level surveys. The spatially correlated variables and logistical considerations that place program villages in close proximity to each other could produce random shocks that yield misleading estimates of program effects. An overlap in treatments within a study area also could make it difficult to isolate the partial effects of any particular treatment. Finally, the absence of detailed follow-up on those leaving a village may make it difficult to measure the full effects of the program, particularly if the program, such as one for educational interventions, affects the opportunities for migration among village residents. The broader geographic scale in panel and cohort studies and the emphasis on migrant follow-up substantially diminish the extent of these problems. The broader scale of panel and cohort studies also permits an assessment of whether there is regional heterogeneity in the treatment effects of various programs and, if so, helps to identifiable possible sources of this heterogeneity.

The discussion in this section has addressed primarily the evaluation of programs at the community level. In some situations, however, the primary concern is to identify the effects of programs on particular individuals. For example, while it may be interesting to know whether the introduction of village-level, small-scale group credit affects fertility or child health in a village, it may be especially interesting to know whether such effects are particularly prevalent among those actually participating in the program. Critical in these contexts is the ability to track individuals over time, and thus some of the limitations discussed above of panel and cohort longitudinal data are diminished. However, in any examination of individual effects there are important issues of selective participation in programs that cannot be approached purely as issues of evaluation.

STRUCTURAL ANALYSIS

Structural analysis as applied to empirical research means a variety of different things to scholars in different disciplines and even to researchers within the same disciplines. For some economists, the term applies only to detailed models incorporating maximizing behavior, which are then fit to data to yield fundamental parameters that capture the underlying preferences, constraints, and information of the relevant actors. For other social scientists, structural analysis refers to a detailed characterization of the underlying data-generating process or the extent to which covariates interact at various levels of aggregation. For the purpose of this paper, however, structural analysis is distinguished from measurement and evaluation in terms of its primary focus on trying to uncover the mechanisms underlying observed outcomes. As such, this definition would include both the above uses of the term as well as an intermediate approach of specifying a behavioral model and drawing out implications of this model for specification and testing, but then relying to the extent possible on estimation of simple linear models.

Organizing a discussion of structural analysis around the issue of different forms of longitudinal data collection is substantially more difficult than doing so for measurement or evaluation. Not only is there more variation in the types of techniques used to extract structural information from longitudinal data than for the other objectives, but also less can be said in general about the suitability of particular types of data to specific methodologies. In short, differences in the suitability of any given form of longitudinal data collection for undertaking structural analysis are greater than the differences in the average suitability of these forms. As a result, the rest of this section focuses on the usefulness of longitudinal data in general and less specifically on the relative merits of the different forms of longitudinal data collection.

A debate is currently under way in the field of empirical economics about the merits of structural analysis as defined here. One view claims that longitudinal data, at least when coupled with sufficient naturally or artificially introduced experimentation, substantially limits the need for structural analysis.[1] In an abstract sense, this may be true—by manipulating the environment of particular individuals and communities and then waiting long enough, one could in principle uncover anything one wished to know about the merits of alternative policies and even fundamental aspects of human behavior. In a practical sense, however, this sentiment is clearly wrong. Given the constraints of time and money as well as the ethical limitations on the treatment of human subjects, structural analysis and longitudinal data are very much complementary. To obtain meaningful and gener-

---

[1] Rosenzweig and Wolpin (2000), in a recent review article for the *Journal of Economic Literature*, characterized and critiqued this perspective.

alizable insight into demographic responses to economic and social conditions, a researcher would have to disentangle alternative potential mechanisms, and this process of disentangling is greatly aided by the presence of longitudinal data.

Nonrandom selection provides a first case in which longitudinal data greatly simplifies structural analysis. Examples of selection include the possibility that participants in a program are not randomly selected from all relevant individuals and the notion that those women giving birth in a particular year do not necessarily constitute a random sample of women. A series of both parametric and nonparametric selection techniques are available for cross-sectional data analysis, but these techniques are dependent on functional form, the presence of variables that influence selection but not outcomes net of selection, the extent of conditional independence, or the availability of discontinuities in program access. Addressing selectivity problems tends to be much more straightforward in the context of longitudinal data.

An example is the question of whether the Matlab family planning program had an impact on child health in the period immediately after the introduction of that program in 1978. The dramatic effects of the program on fertility are well known, but it is less well known that the measured effects of the treatment program on mortality were relatively small until 1982 when an intensive maternal and child health program was increasingly integrated into the treatment area (Menken and Phillips, 1990). But does this lack of a substantial differential in mortality during this period reflect the fact that the intensive family planning services and low-level maternal and child health services had little impact on mortality risk for children? Or does it indicate that there was a change in the composition of births because of the introduction of the treatment program, which offset a pronounced reduction in mortality? Results from Foster (1994) that incorporate maternal fixed effects suggest that the latter interpretation is correct: the estimates indicate that the program led to an approximately 20 percent drop in mortality for the children of a given woman. Because mothers with relatively low risks of child loss were among the first to adopt the family planning program, high-risk mothers were differentially represented among the children born after the introduction of the program, thereby masking the favorable effects of the program on mortality risk when viewed from an aggregate perspective. Through the use of longitudinal data the complex problem of fertility selection can be addressed simply with a minimal imposition of structure.

Nonrandom selection also comes into play in the context of attrition, which was discussed in some detail in the section on measurement. Even if complete follow-up of participants in a panel, cohort, or community study is impossible, it may be possible to at least partly assess the implications of attrition through use of the appropriate longitudinal data. By modeling the process of attrition and determining which baseline features predict the probability of participants leaving the sample, some insight may be gained into the possible biases introduced by nonrandom attrition. In repeated cross-sectional data, for example, the investigator generally does not know which individuals have left a given area, thus limiting the scope for analysis of any selectivity introduced by differential departure from a given region of particular types of individuals.

A second area in which longitudinal data can aid in the identification of underlying mechanisms is in the context of intrahousehold allocation. Researchers interested in testing whether bargaining plays an important role in household decision making have used unearned income that is assignable to spouses as a source of identification (e.g., Thomas, 1990). The premise of this approach is that under the unitary or common-preference model a reallocation of the source of financial resources should not change household allocations net of total income. But nonearned income may be a consequence of unequal household allocation: men who have more control over household decision making may have more control over assets acquired by the household over time and thus have higher nonearned income. Even premarital assets may be related to unobserved (to the researcher) attributes of the partners that also influence household allocations through the process of marital sorting. Thus a correlation between the distribution of unearned income and household allocations net of total income need not imply that the unitary household model must be discarded in favor of a more complex alternative incorporating bargaining.

Analysis of this question of whether control over resources affects household allocations is more palatable, however, if individually allocatable consumption or nutritional data are available over time along with measures of unanticipated shocks to income. Duflo and Udry (2001), for example, use rainfall shocks that differentially affect crops cultivated by men and women to test alternative models of intrahousehold allocation utilizing community-based longitudinal data from rural Côte d'Ivoire. The key insight here is that by following households over time it is possible to control for fixed unobservables governing patterns of behavior within a particular household and thus to mimic relatively closely the effect of exogenously redistributing income within the household from one member to the other with total income held fixed.

Longitudinal data also play a critical role in terms of evaluating interhousehold allocations. In the cross section, for example, it is difficult to distinguish financial transfers between households that are, in effect, fixed regular remittances from those that play an important role in insuring against risk. An examination of how transfers change over time produces direct evidence on this point, however. Longitudinal data also can be used to better understand why insurance-based transfers are likely to be imperfect. Recent game-theoretic models of transfer behavior have suggested that, given the difficulty of writing formal enforceable contracts governing transfer behavior, one should expect transfers to exhibit credit-like aspects in the sense that transfers between two households would be negatively autocorrelated across time. Longitudinal transfer data from panel datasets in South Asia tend to support this conclusion (Foster and Rosenzweig, 2001b).

A fourth area in which structural analysis is aided by the presence of longitudinal data is where there may be important lags between the timing at which a particular program or source of economic change is introduced and the time at which this effect is actually realized. Foster and Rosenzweig (2000), for example, use data on agricultural productivity growth from a national longitudinal panel to examine the extent to which male-female mortality differentials are sensitive to the relative returns to male and female human capital. The authors argue that much of the existing literature, which downplays the potential for economic change to influence sex differences in mortality, is misleading because it focuses on income effects (which may be contemporaneous to any consequent changes in morality differentials) rather than incentive effects, which take years to accrue—for example, the benefits of investing in sons and daughters may not be realized until they marry and set up separate households. Anyone evaluating these incentive effects needs data spanning a considerable period as well as a methodological approach that captures forward-looking behavior on the part of parents.

A fifth area in which longitudinal data is critical for structural analysis is in the evaluation of social or community effects on individual behavior. Clearly articulated by Manski (1993), these reflexive problems raise serious identification issues because of the difficulty of distinguishing between shared random shocks and social influence. By paying careful attention to the nature of likely effects and the processes underlying them, however, a researcher can make some progress in this regard using longitudinal data. Foster and Rosenzweig (1995), for example, modeled social influence about the adoption of new agricultural technologies in green revolution India as a kind of learning-by-doing effect in which previous experience by oneself and one's neighbors increased the profitability and thus the adoption of these new technologies. Critical to the identification of this model is the idea that, net of individual-specific fixed effects, the recent history of price and weather shocks affects the current profitability of new technologies only through its effect on current experience with the new technologies. This source of identification would have been useless in the absence of longitudinal data on planting and profitability.

A key requirement of any analysis of social influence is, of course, tracking the social context of people over time, something that may differ in the different forms of longitudinal studies. Panel data capture a sample of the relevant social network in a particular village. But information on such social networks and community effects in general will necessarily be more limited for those leaving the study area. Cohort studies also provide a sample of the relevant social network within a study's cohorts but provide very limited information on social contacts across cohort lines. Whether this loss is important will depend critically on the nature of the social influence being studied. With their relatively comprehensive coverage, community studies are particularly well suited to comprehensive analysis of social networks. Not only can investigators track the behaviors of most of the community members likely to influence a given person (instead of just a sample as in panel and cohort studies), but they also can ask people to identify other people in the community with whom they have had contact and link data on these nominated community members back to the individual in question. The disadvantage of community studies here, however, is, as discussed in the context of evaluation and measurement, the limited geographic coverage—it may yield relatively little independent variation in social effects across the study population.

SYNTHESIS

Given the variety of ways in which longitudinal data are used, little can be said in general from a methodological perspective about how longitudinal data should be collected. Nonetheless, some common threads seem to run through the cases just cited. A particularly prominent thread is that longitudinal data have a particular role to play when trying to disentangle the relationship between a series of interdependent choices. In selection, this interdependence arises, for example, between giving birth and using maternal and child health services; in transfers, it involves choices made by both sending and receiving households; and in social networks, the behaviors of different individuals are importantly related. The fundamental difficulty with analyzing interrelated choices is that it is difficult to imagine, at least in the cross section, an exercise in which one manipulates one such choice without directly affecting the other. The advantage of longitudinal data is that, given the appropriate history dependence, it may be in fact possible to simulate the desired experiment.

A simple example from economics involving estimation of a conditional demand function may be useful.[2] In a consumer choice problem with three or more goods, it is sometimes desirable to assess how the consumption of one of the goods, say good 2, affects the consumption of one of the other goods, say good 1. More specifically, let us think of good 2 as the health of a child, good 1 as the schooling of a child, and good 3 as other consumption, and let us ask whether increases in child health are likely to result in better school attendance for a given income and prices. From an economic perspective, this effect, if present, is complex—it reflects not only the extent to which better health enhances performance in school but also how parents respond to changes in health by putting fewer (or more) resources into their child's education.

In a simple one-period world, this appears to be an intractable problem: given that health and schooling are chosen simultaneously, any household or community variables that influence health also will influence schooling. To implement, using cross-sectional data, the effect of providing a given child with better health and then observing whether education is influenced, one needs some household or community variables that affect health but does not affect schooling directly. An obvious choice might be the cost of health care, but this is not without difficulty—a change in the cost of health care would indeed affect health, but it also would have a direct effect on schooling net of health by influencing the resources available to the household after health expenses are incurred.

The introduction of multiple periods into the analysis can help solve this problem. If, for example, period 2 health is determined by choices

---

[2]The analytic details for the model are presented in the anex to this paper.

made in period 1, then variation in the period 1 price of health care will influence period 2 health without directly affecting resource availability in period 2 (at least in the absence of savings which, in any case, can be measured directly) and thus will affect schooling only through its effect on health. A change in the period 1 price can thus be used to examine the effect of changing the period 2 health of a child without directly influencing schooling. Thus the introduction of history dependence, coupled with the appropriate longitudinal data, solves what seems to be an inherently intractable problem in the cross section. Longitudinal data therefore allows antecedents of current outcomes to be used to simulate variation in these outcomes and thereby to disentangle the relationships between interdependent choices.

CONCLUSION

Longitudinal data have the potential to substantially increase understanding of human behavior and the impacts of programs and policies. The extent to which this potential is realized varies greatly according to the ways in which the data are collected, the purpose of the analysis, the methodologies employed, the substantive issues being considered, the statistical and survey capacity of the area being examined, and the availability of other data sources in that area. It is not clear that it is desirable to focus data collection in any one particular way. But there does seem to be a need to consider carefully how history dependence is captured in longitudinal data and how this dependence can best be exploited to better understand the mechanisms underlying important demographic outcomes.

ANNEX

Consider a utility function $u(c_{t1}, c_{t2}, c_{t3})$ and a budget constraint $p_{t1}c_{t1} + p_{t2}c_{t2} + p_{t3}c_{t3} = y_t$, where c_{ti} denotes consumption of good i at time t, p_{ti} denotes prices, and y_t denotes income. If the consumer can freely choose levels of consumption of each of the three goods, the choices are interdependent and the relevant demand functions are of the form

(2) $\quad c_{t1} = C_i(p_{t1}, p_{t2}, p_{t3}, y_t)$

Asking the question of how an increase in good 2 affects good 1, however, in effect imposes an additional artificial constraint on the consumer by setting the value of c_{t2} to some level $c_{t2}{}^*$ and then considering the effect of an increase in $c_{t2}{}^*$ on the consumption of good 1. Solving this new problem as one of constrained maximization problem yields a function for c_{t1} that depends on $c_{t2}{}^*$ and on all prices and income so that

(3) $\quad c_{ti} = C_1{}^*(c_{t2}{}^*, p_{t1}, p_{t2}, p_{t3}, y_t)$

This equation looks estimable, in principle, but because the constraint on c_2 is not in fact faced by the consumers, the levels of consumer choice actually observed is fully determined by the arguments to (2), which appear as well in (3). Thus there is no feasible way to change c_{t2} with p_{ti} and y_t fixed—a change in c_{t2} can only come about through a change in one of these other variables.

If good 2 (health) is determined according to the resources and information available in period 0 and cannot otherwise be altered in period 1, then $c_{12} = c_{02}$. The period 0 budget constraint is that just described, but the period 1 budget constraint is

(4) $\quad p_{11}c_{11} + p_{13}c_{13} = y_1$

The unconditional demand for c_{12} will then depend on period 0 and period 1 (to the extent these are known at time 1) prices and income, so that

(5) $\quad c_{12} = C_{12}(p_{01}, p_{02}, p_{03}, y_0, p_{11}, p_{13}, y_1)$

The conditional demand (3) is, however, identical except that p_{12} is omitted:

(6) $\quad c_{11} = c_{11}{}^*(c_{12}{}^*, p_{11}, p_{13}, y_1)$

A comparison of (5) and (6) indicates that the problem arising in (2) and (3) no longer obtains. It is straightforward to imagine an increase in consumption of good 2 in period 1 (as a consequence, say, of changes in period 1 prices) while leaving the other arguments of (6) unchanged.

REFERENCES

Cleland, J., J.F. Phillips, S. Amin, and G.M. Kamal
    1994 *The Determinants of Reproductive Change in Bangladesh: Success in a Challenging Environment.* Washington, DC: World Bank, Regional and Sectoral Studies.

Duflo, E., and C. Udry
    2001 Risk and Intrahousehold Resource Allocation in Côte d'Ivoire. Unpublished manuscript Massachusetts Institute of Technology.

Foster, A.D.
    1994 Program Effects and the Allocation of Resources within the Household. Unpublished manuscript Brown University. Available online at http://adfdell.pstc.brown.edu/papers/gwu.pdf

Foster, A.D., and M.R. Rosenzweig
    1995 Learning by doing and learning from others: Human capital and technical change in agriculture. *Journal of Political Economy* 103(6):1176-1209.
    2000 Missing women, marriage markets, and economic growth. Unpublished manuscript, Brown University. Available online at: *http://adfdell.pstc.brown.edu/papers/sex.pdf*
    2001a Household division, inequality and rural economic growth. *Review of Economic Studies*. Available online at: http://adfdell.pstc.brown.edu/papers/split.pdf
    2001b Imperfect commitment, altruism, and the family: Evidence from transfer behavior in low-income rural areas. *Review of Economics and Statistics* 83(3):389-407 (August).

Gertler, P.J., and J.W. Molyneaux
    1994 How economic-development and family-planning programs combined to reduce Indonesian fertility. *Demography* 31(1):33-63.

Glewwe, P.W., and M. Grosh, eds.
    2000 *Designing Household Survey Questionnaires for Developing Countries: Lessons from 15 Years of the Living Standards Development Study.* New York: Oxford University Press.

Manski, C.F.
    1993 Identification of endogenous social effects—The reflection problem. *Review of Economic Studies* 60(3):531-542.

Menken, J., and J. Phillips
    1990 Demographic change in rural Bangladesh: Evidence from Matlab. *Annals of the American Academy of Political and Social Science* 510:87-101.

Pitt, M.M., M.R. Rosenzweig, and D.M. Gibbons
    1993 The determinants and consequences of the placement of government programs in Indonesia. *World Bank Economic Review* 7(3):319-348.

Pollitt, E., K.S. Gorman, P.L. Engle, J.A. Rivera, and R. Martorell
    1995 Nutrition in early life and the fulfillment of intellectual potential. *Journal of Nutrition* 1125(4 Suppl):1111S-1118S.

Rosenzweig, M.R., and K.I. Wolpin
    1988 Migration selectivity and the effects of public programs. *Journal of Public Economics* 37(3):265-289.

2000 Natural "natural experiments" in economics. *Journal of Economic Literature* 38(4):827-874.

Schultz, T.P.
1973 Explanation of birth rate changes over space and time: A study of Taiwan. *Journal of Political Economy* 81(2, Part 2): S238-S274.

Thomas, D.
1990 Intrahousehold resource allocation: An inferential approach. *Journal of Human Resources* 25(fall):635-664.

Thomas, D., E. Frankenberg, and J.P. Smith
2001 *Lost But Not Forgotten: Attrition in the Indonesian Family Life Survey.* RAND RP-965. RAND, Santa Monica, CA.

Overview of Ethical Issues in Collecting Data in Developing Countries, with Special Reference to Longitudinal Designs

Richard A. Cash and Tracy L. Rabin
Program on Ethical Issues in International Health Research
Department of Population and International Health
Harvard School of Public Health

This paper identifies major ethical issues in longitudinal health research and demographic and health data collection and analysis, specifically as they are related to research conducted in developing countries. A discussion of general ethical principles for health research and questions of community-based ethics is followed by a description of the benefits and risks of longitudinal health research, with special reference to the issues of informed consent, confidentiality, and researcher responsibilities to the host community.

BASIC PRINCIPLES OF ETHICAL RESEARCH

Discussions of biomedical ethics usually begin with the introduction of four basic principles: respect for persons, beneficence, nonmaleficence, and justice. This set of principles was first formalized in the *Belmont Report,* the final product of the U.S. National Commission for the Protection of Human Subjects of Biomedical and Behavioral Research (1979). This commission was charged with identifying the basic ethical principles that should underlie the conduct of biomedical and behavioral research using human subjects and then developing guidelines to ensure that such research is conducted in accordance with the basic principles.

Since the release of the *Belmont Report,* the import of these four principles has become recognized internationally. As a set of key considerations in the design and implementation of ethical research, however, they are by no means all-encompassing, and additional principles have been articulated in the literature. Contending that good scientific research is not necessarily ethical research, Emanuel et al. (2000) recently proposed a set of seven requirements to ensure that clinical research is ethical: (1) social or scientific value; (2) scientific validity; (3) fair subject selection; (4) favorable risk/benefit ratio; (5) independent review; (6) informed consent; and (7) respect for potential and enrolled subjects. Each of these principles also applies to community-based studies and data collection and requires that community needs and values be considered along with those of the individual.

In September 2000, the Indian Council on Medical Research (ICMR) published *Ethical Guidelines for Biomedical Research on Human Subjects*, an excellent example of a high-quality developing country document (Indian Council on Medical Research, 2000). The ICMR proposed that 12 general principles be considered in designing research projects involving human subjects: (1) essentiality (of the research); (2) voluntariness, informed consent, and community agreement; (3) nonexploitation; (4) privacy and confidentiality; (5) precaution and risk minimization; (6) professional competence; (7) accountability and transparency; (8) maximization of the public interest and of distributive justice; (9) institutional arrangements; (10) public domain; (11) totality of responsibility; and (12) compliance.

These sets of formally articulated ethical principles cover a wide spectrum, ranging from (but not limited to) the four broad principles of the Belmont Report to the more specific set of twelve principles provided by the ICMR. The variation in the items on these lists demonstrates that no single list of principles has authority over others, although some are cited more often. It is instructive to examine the application of these principles in the context of the different international guidelines that have been published over the past 40 years.

INTERNATIONAL GUIDELINES

Worldwide, several documents have been formulated to provide researchers with a standard set of directions for ensuring that the human subjects of their research are "adequately" protected.[1] An early document,

---

[1] Here "adequate" protection is equivalent to the level of human subject protection that is considered appropriate under the internationally recognized guidelines.

the *Nuremberg Code,* emerged from the 1949 "Trials of War Criminals before the Nuremberg Military Tribunals" as a direct reaction to the crimes perpetrated by German doctors against human research subjects during the Nazi regime (U.S. Government Printing Office, 1949). This 10-point document deals primarily with the idea that acceptable consent to participate in research is an irrevocable requirement and can only be given voluntarily and by persons who "have sufficient knowledge and comprehension of the elements of the subject matter involved as to enable him to make an understanding and enlightened decision" (U.S. Government Printing Office, 1949). Though the German doctors have been held up as the ultimate example of unethical treatment of human subjects, the Japanese Imperial Army's Unit 731 was responsible for similar atrocities against the Chinese in World War II. Unlike the German doctors in the trials at Nuremberg, however, many of the Japanese perpetrators were released by the U.S. Army in exchange for their data.

The World Medical Association, founded in 1947 as an independent confederation of medical associations worldwide, adopted the *Declaration of Helsinki* as its organizational policy on ethical principles for medical research involving human subjects in 1964 (World Medical Assembly, 1964). This document was, historically, the follow-up to the *Nuremberg Code,* although it was intended primarily to govern physician-researchers, not researchers in general. The *Declaration of Helsinki* is not itself a legally binding document, and it has undergone five revisions since it was first adopted. The most recent revision was adopted in October 2000 and is composed of 32 standalone clauses (World Medical Association, 2000). The *Declaration* has been used to inform World Health Organization (WHO) practices and national legislation in various countries.

The Council for International Organizations of Medical Sciences (CIOMS) is an international, nongovernmental, not-for-profit organization that was jointly established by WHO and the United Nations Educational, Scientific, and Cultural Organization (UNESCO) in 1949. CIOMS has three main objectives: (1) facilitating and promoting international activities in the field of biomedical sciences; (2) maintaining collaborative relations with the United Nations and its specialized agencies; and (3) serving the scientific interests of the international biomedical community in general. In 1991, after two years of international discussion, CIOMS published the *International Guidelines for Ethical Review of Epidemiological Studies* (Council for International Organizations of Medical Sciences, 1991). These guidelines are designed to aid in the development of national policies on the ethics of epidemiological research and practice and the ethical review of epidemiological studies. They are intended for all people (not just physicians) who face the ethical issues that arise in the course of epidemiological research, including scientific investigators, health policy-makers, and ethical review committee members.

The *International Ethical Guidelines for Biomedical Research Involving Human Subjects* (Council for International Organizations of Medical Sciences, 1993), originally published by CIOMS in 1993 and presently undergoing revisions, replaced a 1982 set of proposed guidelines that were intended to elucidate how to apply effectively the ethical principles set forth in the *Declaration of Helsinki*, with particular attention to research conducted in developing countries. The *International Ethical Guidelines for Biomedical Research Involving Human Subjects* are designed for use in developing national policies on ethical biomedical research and mechanisms for ethical review of research using human subjects. In addition to recognizing the importance of both clinical and nonclinical research, the preamble to the guidelines contains an extensive list of the various types of research that fall under the category of "research involving human subjects."

In April 2001, the U.S. National Bioethics Advisory Commission (NBAC) published a report entitled *Ethical and Policy Issues in International Research: Clinical Trials in Developing Countries—Volume I, Report and Recommendations of the National Bioethics Advisory Commission* (U.S. National Bioethics Advisory Commission, 2001). The purpose of this document is to respond to ethical issues that arise over the course of research in developing countries that is subject to U.S. regulation. Although the recommendations contained in the report can be applied to many types of research, the scope of this document was mainly limited to issues related to clinical trials involving competent adult participants.

DEFINING THE COMMUNITY AND COMMUNITY-BASED ETHICS

As longitudinal research requires that human subjects be considered at both the community level and individual level, special conditions affect ethical concerns for the community. The community-level concerns include: how to obtain communal approval; potential benefits and risks to groups with varying literacy levels; use of incentives; the issue of providing feedback and results to the host community; and anonymity of communities. Until recently, these concerns had not been directly addressed in an official document, although several of the documents described earlier in this paper now contain guidelines that can be extended to community-based research.

The *International Guidelines for Ethical Review of Epidemiological Studies* published by CIOMS acknowledges in Guideline 25 that there are often cultural differences between researchers and research subjects:

> Investigators must respect the ethical standards of their own countries and the cultural expectations of the societies in which epidemiological studies are undertaken, unless this implies a violation of a transcending moral rule. Investigators risk harming their reputation by pursuing work that host countries find acceptable but their own countries consider offensive. Similarly, they may transgress the cultural values of the host countries by uncritically conforming to the expectations of their own. (Council for International Organizations of Medical Sciences, 1991)

This statement provides little actual guidance, however, about how these differences can be handled in an ethical fashion, other than making the claim that a set of (unidentified) "transcendent" moral rules exist.

A community may be thought of as "a group of people understood as having a certain identity due to the sharing of common interests, a common set of values, a common disease or a shared geographical proximity" (Weijer and Emanuel, 2000). In demographic health research or evaluation projects, however, communities are much more narrowly defined. Focusing on one particular community or group of people serves to decrease the cost of the study and potentially increase the quality of the data collected over time (follow-up is easier). These are especially important considerations in areas that do not have reliable health or demographic data registration systems. Depending on the research topic or the results of the study, however, the focus on one community may lead to stigmatization or discrimination by its neighbors or within the larger society. The tension between defining a community for research purposes and minimizing the potential social harms associated with being identified with such a group is an important concern. In addition, individuals are usually members of several different communities simultaneously, depending on the definition of a community. Therefore, one community could benefit from the involvement of some of its members in a research project, whereas another community (of which some of those same individuals are members) could be affected in a negative way.

To minimize the potential risks to host communities, some questions must be addressed before identifying a group. Is a particular population potentially overrepresented in a study, so that it might appear that the condition under investigation is more prevalent in that group? How are potential participants approached or selected? Can the findings be generalized to a larger community, and is it scientifically valid to do so? Coughlin notes:

> Epidemiological research does not take place in a social vacuum, and areas of ethical conflict may exist between the need to obtain scientifically accurate information about the health of population subgroups and the moral imperative to avoid harming populations that already suffer stigmatization and discrimination from the mainstream societies in which they live. (Coughlin, 1996)

The type of community-based research conducted is an extension of concerns about the definition of a host community. The draft revision of the CIOMS *International Ethical Guidelines for Biomedical Research Involving Human Subjects* offers two statements in response to this question. Guideline 6 states that the research should be "responsive to the health needs and the priorities of the population or community in which it is to be carried out" (Council for International Organizations of Medical Sciences, 2001). This is similar to Principle 19 in the most recent revision of the *Declaration of Helsinki,* which asserts that "medical research is only justified if there is a reasonable likelihood that the populations in which the research is carried out stand to benefit from the results of the research" (World Medical Assembly, 2000). These comments were added, it seems, to ensure that research in developing countries (especially that sponsored by institutions or industry from developed countries) not be conducted there simply because of lower costs or absent or slack regulations. The dilemma is how does one determine "reasonable likelihood"?

Research should first address local needs. When initially tested in developing countries, the hepatitis B vaccine was priced way beyond their reach. Hepatitis B was, however, a local problem, and the price has now come down to a level that allows the vaccine to be used widely in many countries, especially in East and Southeast Asia. Given that the vaccine was initially unaffordable to the majority of Chinese citizens, should it not have been tested in China? This also raises the question of what to do if a government refuses to distribute an effective product within the national health care system, such as the South African government's refusal to distribute nevirapine to HIV/AIDS patients. Does this mean that no studies involving that product can be conducted in that country? Should the researcher be held responsible for the government policy? As official government positions and policies are constantly changing, this hardly seems to be a sensible recommendation.

There is also the matter of how involved host communities should be in setting the research agenda and to what degree community representatives should be involved in study design or in deciding how to use collected data. Recommendation 2.3 of the NBAC report *Ethical and Policy Issues in International Research* calls for the involvement of host community representatives in the entire development and implementation of research projects. If community representatives decline to be involved in the processes, investigators are required to justify this to their ethical review committee(s) (U.S. National Bioethics Advisory Commission, 2001). The rationale for recommending this level of community involvement is that these consultations will provide a greater insight into the relevance of the research question(s) to the host community and may better inform the development of the consent process. Increased community involvement marks a dramatic shift in the historically paternalistic attitudes of many researchers, serving to improve the relationship between investigators and the host community.

ISSUES OF INFORMED CONSENT

Informed consent is the primary ethical concern of many researchers and ethical review boards (ERBs). All international guidelines consider consent "informed" if the participant knows the purpose and nature of the study, the nature of his or her participation, and the potential risks and benefits involved. Implicit in this definition, however, is the belief that potential participants will understand the information they are given. Today, the practice of obtaining informed consent has become a matter of following more the letter than the spirit of the law. Perhaps the requirements should direct researchers to obtain "understood" consent—confirmation that participants understand what they are consenting to—rather than simply document that the conversation took place.

At present, most guidelines deal specifically with obtaining consent from individuals (and express a strong preference for written proof of consent), because this method traditionally has been used by researchers in the developed world. When dealing with less educated populations (in both developed and developing countries), however, researchers may find it difficult to explain sufficiently the purpose, benefits, and potential risks of a study. Moreover, written consent forms are not always appropriate for illiterate populations or for particular social, political, or cultural traditions. The ICMR *Ethical Guidelines for Biomedical Research on Human Subjects* address these issues, acknowledging that many communities in India, because of an insufficient level of education, are less able to understand study procedures or implications than communities in more developed countries:

> When individuals are to be the subject of any epidemiological studies, the purpose and general objectives of the study has to be explained to them keeping in mind their level of understanding. . . . In the context of developing countries, obtaining informed consent has been considered many times as difficult/impractical/not meeting the purpose on various grounds such as incompetence to comprehend the meaning or relevance of the consent. . . . [H]owever, **there is no alternative to obtaining individual's informed consent** but what should be the content of the informed consent is also a crucial issue. (Indian Council on Medical Research, 2000; emphasis in original)

One of the contentious issues that has surfaced in some countries is whether it is ethically acceptable for a representative of the community to give consent for individual members of the community. This issue is addressed in Guideline 5 of the CIOMS *International Guidelines for Ethical Review of Epidemiological Studies*:

> When it is not possible to request informed consent from every individual to be studied, the agreement of a representative of a community or group may be sought, but the representative should be chosen according to the nature, traditions, and political philosophy of the community or group. . . . For communities in which collective decision-making is customary, communal leaders can express the collective will. However, the refusal of individuals to participate in a study has to be respected; a leader may express agreement on behalf of a community but an individual's refusal of personal participation is binding. (Council for International Organizations of Medical Sciences, 1991)

The consent of other parties is also involved in many other situations—that is, other than those requiring collective decision-making. For example, in some cultures women traditionally cannot provide their own consent, or a woman's husband or father must grant his permission before she can consent to participate in research. Recognizing that these situations are generally one-sided (meaning that women generally are in the position of needing a man's permission), NBAC Recommendation 3.9 states:

> Researchers should use the same procedures in the informed consent process for women and men. However, ethics review committees may accept a consent process in which a woman's individual consent to participate in research is supplemented by permission from a man if all of the following conditions

> are met: . . . it would be impossible to conduct the research without obtaining such supplemental permission; and...failure to conduct this research would deny its potential benefits to women in the host country; and . . . measures to respect the woman's autonomy to consent in research are undertaken to the greatest extent possible. In no case may a competent adult woman be enrolled in research solely upon the consent of another person; her individual consent is always required. (U.S. National Bioethics Advisory Commission, 2001)

The three special conditions under which supplemental permission is acceptable are written with the intent of protecting researchers' abilities to conduct research around issues that affect only women and to ensure that the women would not be denied benefits that can only result from such research (e.g., the information needed to list women's health care needs by priority in that population).

Dealing with informed consent in a longitudinal study also presents a number of other issues. For example, if the subjects are "minors" (and the definition may well be culturally dependent) at the outset of the study and will become adults over the course of the follow-up period, does consent for participation have to be obtained twice? Should consent for a long-term longitudinal study that goes on for years ever have to be renegotiated and, if so, how often? How long after a study is completed should investigators be responsible for returning to the community to share data and make recommendations? Should a follow-up period be scheduled to maximize the benefits that might accrue from the delivery of health care in the community as compared with the potential risks to the individual? In addition, when dealing with biological specimens that have been collected and stored over a period of time are researchers required to seek additional consent from participants in order to conduct additional research on those materials? The NBAC report *Research Involving Human Biological Materials: Ethical Issues and Policy Guidance* provides an elaborate discussion of guidelines for collecting specimens for storage, testing, and later use (U.S. National Bioethics Advisory Commission, 1999).

Questions about the appropriateness of obtaining re-consent for research are dealt with in the CIOMS draft revision of the *International Ethical Guidelines for Biomedical Research Involving Human Subjects*. Addressing the planning and initial stages of research, the commentary on Guideline 9 states:

> All individuals enrolled as research subjects should be allowed to decide about potential uses of their biological materials for research. . . . Subjects

should be told whether the specimens will be stored for future research, and, if so, for how long, and whether the nature of the future research is currently unknown, whether the materials will be shared with other researchers, and whether commercial products will be developed from the specimens. (Council for International Organizations of Medical Sciences, 2001)

This passage suggests that participants would decide from the outset whether they consent to future research using their specimens or information. While this advance planning may prevent some problems for future research, it is not difficult to imagine a situation in which an ethical review committee does not accept (as "informed consent for future research") the fact that participants were told at the outset that research might be conducted at some point in the future. The last three sentences of this commentary are particularly relevant to the use of medical records in research, requiring that

> [p]atients should be told about the possible research uses of their medical records and of biological specimens that are taken in the course of clinical care. In many cases it will suffice to notify patients that research involving such records or specimens is commonly performed without individual informed consent. In other cases, the research ethics committee may require individual informed consent. (Council for International Organizations of Medical Sciences, 2001)

This section raises interesting questions about the role of local medical practitioners in research. For studies involving data from medical records, should all physicians have to explain to patients that their medical records may be used for research purposes, even if their anonymity is maintained? This is an important question, considering the potential for negative effects on health-care-seeking behavior. Is it even appropriate for physicians to be in the position of having to explain the concepts of "research" and "informed consent" to their patients? The notion of research does not exist or is very poorly understood in many cultures. Where records are unlinked or delinked and the risk to the individual is minimal or nonexistent, the local ethical review board should determine whether informed consent is required.

The commentary on Guideline 10 of the CIOMS draft revision provides some guidance for questions of re-consent that may arise after the initial stages of the research:

> Medical records and biological specimens may be used for research without the consent of the patients/subjects only if an ethics review board has decided that the protocol poses minimal risk, that the rights or interests of the pa-

tients will not be violated, and that the research is designed to answer an important question and could not practicably be conducted with specimens and records for which informed consent had been obtained.... Records and specimens of individuals who have specifically rejected such uses in the past may be used only in the case of public health emergencies. (Council for International Organizations of Medical Sciences, 2001)

Thus, according to the CIOMS, the ultimate decision about whether re-consent is required should fall on the shoulders of the ethical review committee(s). This external check on researchers' activities serves to satisfy the requirement in the *Declaration of Helsinki* that "[e]very precaution should be taken to respect the privacy of the subject and the confidentiality of the patient's information" (World Medical Assembly, 2000).

As part of the informed consent process, a form or script providing the necessary information about the study should be read by or read to the potential participants. What should be the scope of this consent document? If the document is too broad, researchers run the risk of including more information than potential participants need to be able to make an informed decision, or information that is too technically involved for participants to understand. But if the document is too limited, researchers run the risk of not including enough of the information potential participants need to be able to make an informed decision. Another problem is how to communicate the necessary information when the population of interest is illiterate.

Finally, in light of the recent shift toward an increased emphasis on the informed consent process, how should the investigator determine whether the participant truly understands the potential risks, benefits, and procedures of the study? Researchers will likely approach such a question differently if understanding becomes the focus of the process. The NBAC report *Ethical and Policy Issues in International Research: Clinical Trials in Developing Countries* provides a more detailed discussion of this issue (U.S. National Bioethics Advisory Commission, 2001).

ISSUES OF CONFIDENTIALITY

Personal information collected by researchers may be damaging to either individuals or a community if disclosed to a third party. Stigmatization, discrimination, and other social or physical harms may occur if participants in a study are identified as different in some way from a larger community. Investigators must be able to assure participants that all information collected will be protected and, where appropriate, will not be linked to an individual or a group or community. Depending on the research topic, participation in a study itself may have to be treated in a confidential manner (e.g., vaginal microbicide trials or tests of family planning methods).

When information collected as part of a study is not linked to an individual or community (i.e., it is collected anonymously or without personal identifiers), breach of confidentiality is not a concern. Longitudinal research raises special issues, however, because it may be necessary to maintain a linkage between data and identifying variables for the purpose of collecting follow-up information. These data are termed "confidential"—information that is collected using either personal identifiers (and then is kept in a storage facility with strictly controlled access) or using unique identifiers that are associated with a key (also stored under secure conditions) to allow matching of individuals or groups with the identifiers. Because researchers working on longitudinal studies expect a certain number of participants to be "lost to follow-up" (and will try to minimize this number), consideration must be given early on to how to minimize this loss within the context of maintaining confidentiality. In addition, investigators need to consider issues of confidentiality along with the question of potential obligations to track participants down and notify them of any unanticipated study results that may have personal implications.

Due to the risks involved in using data that have explicit personal identifiers, investigators should justify to the ERB the need for linked data and provide a detailed explanation of how confidentiality will be protected. Regardless, communities (and individuals) may want to remain anonymous if the disclosure of research findings could potentially harm the community. For example, a high prevalence of a particular disease in a community or occupational group, such as the prevalence of HIV/AIDS among commercial sex workers, may stigmatize the group. The CIOMS *International Guidelines for Ethical Review of Epidemiological Studies* address the issues related to "harmful publicity" in Guideline 22:

> Conflict may appear between, on the one hand, doing no harm and, on the other, telling the truth and openly disclosing scientific findings. Harm may be mitigated by interpreting data in a way that protects the interests of those at risk, and is at the same time consistent with scientific integrity. Investigators should, where possible, anticipate and avoid misinterpretation that might cause harm. (Council for International Organizations of Medical Sciences, 1991)

These statements presume that investigators are in the best position to make judgments about the best way to prevent harm. As suggested in the NBAC report (U.S. National Bioethics Advisory Commission, 2001), however, there may be a role for community representatives at this stage of the research project, because they could provide important insight into how to minimize potential harms. In the interest of full disclosure of potential harms, the commentary on Guideline 19 of the draft revision of the *International Ethical Guidelines for Biomedical Research Involving Human Subjects* requires that information about the efforts that will be taken to ensure confidentiality be included in the informed consent process and, just as important, that prospective research participants "be informed of limits to the researchers' ability to ensure strict confidentiality and of the foreseeable adverse social consequences of breaches of confidentiality" (Council for International Organizations of Medical Science, 2001).

In light of these concerns, it is also important to raise questions about who should ultimately have the power to decide about the publication of certain data, and whether the host community should have a say in the matter (and, if yes, to what extent). Data sharing is important to the demographic community (and the general scientific community), producing tension between the desire to improve general knowledge of the long-term effects of various factors on individuals and populations and the desire of research subjects to have control over information about their private lives. This tension requires balancing two legitimate interests: transparency for the sake of science and concealment of information out of respect for subjects. Important questions stem from this conflict, including deciding who should have access to certain information and who should have the right to agree or disagree to have that information used for various purposes. The answers to these questions stem from the solution to the underlying question: What are the obligations of the data collectors to the persons who are registered in the database?

The CIOMS *International Guidelines for Ethical Review of Epidemiological Studies* address the investigators' responsibilities in Guideline 21:

> Investigators who find sensitive information that may put a group at risk of adverse criticism or treatment should be discreet in communication and the explanation of their findings. When the location or circumstances of a study are important to understanding the results the investigators must explain by what means they propose to protect the group from harm or disadvantage; such means include provisions for confidentiality and the use of language

that does not imply moral criticism of subjects' behavior. (Council for International Organizations of Medical Sciences, 1991)

Although the clause requiring investigators to "explain" proposed means to protect against harm does not explicitly state the identity of the "explainee," it would seem appropriate that the means of protection be explained to the host community (to reach a consensus on the importance of disclosure). It also might be appropriate to justify the disclosure of identifying information to an ethical review board. This step, however, is not common practice as part of preparing research results for publication and, if anticipated, could be better addressed in the initial application for ethical review committee approval.

OBLIGATIONS TO RESEARCH PARTICIPANTS

Individual participants in a study seldom receive many direct benefits or, in some cases, benefits may be difficult to quantify. In a phase I drug trial, for example, the potential benefits to the individual are few. For nonintervention studies, the community benefits may not be as tangible to each individual as the more traditional benefits (such as new jobs related to the research project, a new clinic, and information for subjects about their health status and health risks), or they may be time-limited (such as— during the study—additional health care and improved access to drugs or procedures that have a direct effect on health). More sustainable modes of compensation (such as strengthening health data management capacity or training local staff) may be more appropriate, however. Increased economic activity surrounding a research project, including the use and purchase of equipment, and the construction of new buildings, is also an important benefit.

The draft revision of the CIOMS guidelines and the recently released NBAC report have given more attention to the responsibilities of the researcher to the community than other guidelines (Helsinki) or earlier CIOMS guidelines. They are concerned with what happens within the relationship between the researcher and the research subjects at the conclusion of the study: What should be provided to research participants and by whom? What, if anything, should be made available to others in the host community or country?

Guideline 6 in the draft revision of the 1993 CIOMS *International Ethical Guidelines for Biomedical Research Involving Human Subjects* states:

> Before undertaking research in a population or community with limited resources, the sponsor and the researcher must make every effort to ensure that . . . the research is responsive to the health needs and the priorities of the community in which it is to be carried out . . . and . . . any product developed will be made reasonably available to that population or community. (Council for International Organizations of Medical Sciences, 2001)

What is meant by "reasonable" and "available"? Should the "population" only include those persons involved in the research, or should it also include the geographic region, a particular group of people, or the entire country?

The commentary goes on to interpret the notion of responsiveness as more than simply confirming that a particular health problem is prevalent in a community. It calls for successful interventions developed during the research or any other beneficial research conclusions to be made available to the population. CIOMS recommends that these arrangements be negotiated before the research begins and that a variety of host community and country representatives be involved in this process.

As for negotiating the post-project researcher-participant relationship, NBAC Recommendation 4.1 makes a similar suggestion:

> Researchers and sponsors in the clinical trials should make reasonable, good faith efforts before the initiation of a trial to secure, at its conclusion, continued access for all participants to needed experimental interventions that have been proven effective for the participants. . . . R]esearch protocols should typically describe the duration, extent, and financing of such continued access. When no arrangements have been negotiated, the researcher should justify to the ethics review committee why this is the case. (U.S. National Bioethics Advisory Commission, 2001)

These requirements are less extreme than the controversial clause in the most recent version of the *Declaration of Helsinki,* which states: "At the conclusion of the study, every patient entered into the study should be assured of access to the best proven prophylactic, diagnostic and therapeutic methods identified by the study" (World Medical Assembly, 2000). If upheld, the mandate that investigators provide their participants with access to the best proven intervention—which often far exceeds the community standard of care and is likely to be unsustainable over the long term—may limit the types of research that can be conducted in the developing country context beyond the exploitative situations that the mandate is meant to prevent. Most research in developing countries is, after all, locally funded. As written, the guideline implies immediate access, though such success may not be possible or desirable. This recommendation seems reserved for developing countries. Why adopt this paternalistic approach? Why should local ERBs not make these decisions?

Although most of the international guidelines focus on clinical studies, the principles expressed are relevant to longitudinal studies. If one thinks about collecting information, as opposed to testing interventions, the tie to the longitudinal studies becomes clear. But should all information be released to the individual participants or the host community? What if the release of information to certain groups puts other groups at increased risk of harm? For example, a study of sexual behavior may reveal unexpectedly high rates of extramarital affairs among the women. Would it be ethical for the information to be released to the men of the community if it puts the women at risk?

Just because an intervention has proven to be effective in a developing country context does not mean it is appropriate to release it in the developed world or other communities in the developing world. A drug or vaccine should first be adequately studied in a setting similar to that in which it would be used. The surveillance systems of most poor countries are usually inadequate to detect all but the most obvious side effects of a drug or vaccine.

Regardless of the specific type of research being conducted or the exact location, clearly greater attention should be paid to issues at the community level. Michael Bennish, director of the Africa Centre for Health and Population Studies (KwaZulu Natal, South Africa) states at the conclusion of a video case study dealing with questions of researcher responsibilities to the community:

> We certainly have relatively well-defined policies for ethical conduct of research as it affects an individual. There are far fewer guidelines, and certainly much less in the way of specifics, that deal with the obligation of a research program to communities at large. (John F. Kennedy School of Government Case Program, 1999)

As a related issue, Guideline 22 of the draft revision of the *International Ethical Guidelines for Biomedical Research Involving Human Subjects* deals with the approval of externally sponsored research:

> An external sponsoring agency should submit the research protocol to ethical and scientific review in the country of the sponsoring agency and according to the standards of that country, and the ethical standards applied should be no less exacting than they would be for research carried out in that country. Appropriate authorities of the host country, including a national or local

ethical review committee or its equivalent, should ensure that the proposed research meets their own ethical standards. (Council for International Organizations of Medical Sciences, 2001)

This statement does not offer specific solutions to conflicts between ethical review authorities in the sponsoring and host countries. The guideline does specify, however, that the host country committees are responsible for determining whether the research objectives are responsive to the needs and priorities of the country, and charges ethical reviewers in the sponsoring countries with the task of ensuring compliance with broad ethical standards. This guideline suggests that it is unethical to conduct research in a particular country if the study in question would not receive the approval of the ethical review board of the sponsoring agency. The guideline is a version of a more extreme guideline that appeared in the 1993 draft of the document. It stated that investigators working in less developed communities "must ensure that ... persons in underdeveloped communities will not ordinarily be involved in research that could be carried out reasonably well in developed communities" (Council for International Organizations of Medical Sciences, 1993).

FUTURE DIRECTIONS

Future ethical concerns will be influenced by factors that bear on the types of research questions that investigators will be able to ask, including rapid advancements in the fields of genomics and biotechnology. In addition, developing country governments and institutions will continue to make their voices heard as they become more equal partners in the international research community and as the need for formal training around ethical issues continues to grow.

Genomics and Biotechnology

Science and technology are advancing faster than the ability of the scientific community to handle the moral and ethical dilemmas produced by such advances. Longitudinal studies have faced some of these issues in genetics research and the storing of biologic specimens. Developing countries will exert more pressure to retain some degree of ownership of biologic specimens collected for research purposes, and they will increasingly focus on securing access to benefits that result from research projects conducted in their own communities. How much control should a nation-state or a community exercise over a study if the individual participants fully consent to their involvement? Are some of the guidelines that were intended to protect individual research subjects and host communities hindering the process of investigation (and at the expense of those the researchers are trying to assist)?

Capacity for Ethical Review in Developing Countries

U.S. guidelines insist that the institutions or countries in which research will take place have the capability to conduct their own independent ethical reviews. With the exception of a handful of ethical review boards in a small number of developing countries, not many meet the standards set forth in these guidelines. Few members of developing country ERBs have had any formal training in research ethics (not unlike IRB members in U.S. institutions), and in many of the ERBs the structure of the review process would not meet the criteria for conducting ethical review of research proposals in most U.S. universities. But this inequality is changing with the development of courses, workshops, and fellowships designed to provide short- and long-term training to researchers and ethical review board members from developing countries. Two such training programs are run through the Program on Ethical Issues in International Health Research at the Harvard School of Public Health, and the Bioethics Institute at the Johns Hopkins University. The UNDP (United Nations Development Programme)-UNFPA (United Nations Population Fund)-WHO-World Bank Special Programme of Research, Development, and Research Training in Human Reproduction, within the WHO Department of Reproductive Health and Research, began conducting capacity-building workshops in 1997 (Thailand) and is continuing to improve capacity in this area. The Joint United Nations Programme on HIV/AIDS (UNAIDS) also has conducted similar workshops in Brazil, India, and South Africa. Most recently, the UNDP-World Bank-WHO Special Programme for Research and Training in Tropical Diseases (TDR) developed programs to increase the capacity for conducting ethical reviews of research in Asian and Western Pacific countries through the Forum for Ethical Review Committees in Asia and the Western Pacific (FERCAP). Similar forums have been held in other regions. The *TDR/WHO Operational Guidelines for Ethics Committees that Review Biomedical Research* (UNDP-World Bank-WHO Special Programme for Research and Training in Tropical Diseases, 2000), designed to define the role and composition of an ethics committee, lay out the requirements for submitting an application for review and detail the review procedure and decision-making process. The guidelines were published in 2000 and have been translated into more than twelve languages.

As these capacity-building efforts increase, developing country scientists are asking that some of the international guidelines be reviewed, giving greater consideration to the situation that exists in these countries. Indeed, many scientists, ERB members, and others have noted informally that much of the research in developing countries does not involve collaboration with Western scientists or companies, and that the international guidelines developed to protect the disadvantaged from foreign exploitation may in fact prevent scientists in developing countries from conducting some research that would, by most standards, be considered ethical in their country (personal communications with participants of research ethics workshops in Mexico, South Africa, India, Pakistan, and Nigeria).

In addition, there is the issue of financial support for developing country ethical review boards. The Partners Human Research Committee, the institutional review board network of the Partners HealthCare System that is affiliated with Harvard University, employs more than 30 persons (not including volunteer committee members) and has a yearly budget in the millions of dollars. By contrast, ERBs in most developing country institutions do not have a budget or staff, and ERB members, many on low university salaries often supplemented by private medical practice, volunteer their time. Most developing country ethical review boards usually have a much smaller workload than U.S. institutional review boards, yet there are still costs associated with time, copying, and transport, among other things. One possible solution is for ERBs to charge a fee to review research proposals—either a flat fee or a percentage of the proposed budget. In addition, outside investigators could consider providing support for the general training of ERB members at collaborating institutions.

With few exceptions, local ERBs will not have all the relevant expertise (i.e., biostatisticians, geneticists, and other experts) to evaluate each and every protocol and will have to seek guidance from elsewhere. Both field scientists and ethicists should be encouraged to support and use Web-based forums for the discussion of ethical dilemmas. One example is the Web site and Listserv administered and maintained by the Program on Ethical Issues in International Health Research at the Harvard School of Public Health (*http://www.hsph.harvard.edu/bioethics*). The Web site, which has been functioning since 1999, serves as a source of general information on the ethics of international health research and a discussion site for research ethics concerns. The Listserv has been operational since the spring of 2000, and the entire discussion (including dialogues on specific case studies and the revisions of the *Declaration of Helsinki* and the 1999 and 2001 NBAC reports) is archived on the Web site. To ensure the success of these resources and the advancement of good science, however, scientists and ethicists have to be open to sharing their expertise.

Following the trends in scientific advancements, ethical issues in health research, especially those relevant to developing countries, will continue to change. Although differences in the recommendations presented in the international guidelines may at times be confusing to the individual investigator, they reflect the fluid nature of this international dialogue. It is important for researchers to remember that the ultimate goal of these guidelines is to improve, not encumber, both the ethical and scientific standards of health research. In the end, each institution will have to apply these guidelines within its local context. These discussions will strengthen the ethical reviews in developing countries and their position as contributors to the global dialogue on research ethics.

REFERENCES

Coughlin, S.S.
    1996 Ethically optimized study designs in epidemiology. In *Ethics and Epidemiology*, S.S. Coughlin and T.L. Beauchamp, eds. New York: Oxford University Press.

Council for International Organizations of Medical Sciences
    1991 *International Guidelines for Ethical Review of Epidemiological Studies.* Geneva: CIOMS.
    1993 *International Ethical Guidelines for Biomedical Research Involving Human Subjects.* Geneva: CIOMS.
    2001 Draft Revision of 1993 *International Ethical Guidelines for Biomedical Research Involving Human Subjects.* Geneva: CIOMS. Available: http://www.cioms.ch [May 30, 2001].

Emanuel, E., D. Wendler, and C. Grady
    2000 What makes clinical research ethical? *JAMA* 283(20):2701-2711.

Indian Council on Medical Research
    2000 *Ethical Guidelines for Biomedical Research on Human Subjects.* New Delhi: ICMR.

John F. Kennedy School of Government Case Program
    1999 Good Neighbors? The Africa Centre and the Local Community in Rural KwaZulu/Natal, South Africa. Videocassette.

UNDP-World Bank-WHO Special Programme for Research and Training in Tropical Diseases (TDR)
    2000   *Operational Guidelines for Ethics Committees that Review Biomedical Research.* Geneva: World Health Organization.

U.S. Government Printing Office
    1949   *The Nuremberg Code.* [Reprinted from *Trials of War Criminals before the Nuremberg Military Tribunals under Control Council Law* 10(2):181-182.] Washington, DC: U.S. Government Printing Office. Available: http://ohsr.od.nih.gov/nuremberg.php3 [June 15, 2001].

U.S. National Bioethics Advisory Commission
    1999   *Research Involving Human Biological Materials: Ethical Issues and Policy Guidance—Volume I, Report and Recommendations of the National Bioethics Advisory Commission.* Available: http://bioethics.georgetown.edu/nbac/hbm.pdf [February 1, 2002].
    2001   *Ethical and Policy Issues in International Research: Clinical Trials in Developing Countries—Volume I, Report and Recommendations of the National Bioethics Advisory Commission.* Available: http://bioethics.georgetown.edu/nbac/clinical/Vol1.pdf [February 2002].

U.S. National Commission for the Protection of Human Subjects of Biomedical and Behavioral Research
    1979   *The Belmont Report: Office of the Secretary. Ethical Principles and Guidelines for the Protection of Human Subjects of Research.* Available: http://ohrp.osophs.dhhs.gov/humansubjects/guidance/Belmont.htm [May 7, 2001].

Weijer, C., and E.J. Emanuel
    2000   Protecting communities in biomedical research. *Science* 289:1142-1144.

World Medical Assembly
    1964   *World Medical Association Declaration of Helsinki: Ethical Principles for Medical Research Involving Human Subjects.* 1st ed. Helsinki: 18th World Medical Assembly.
    2000   *World Medical Association Declaration of Helsinki: Ethical Principles for Medical Research Involving Human Subjects.* 6th ed. Edinburgh: 52nd World Medical Assembly. Available: http://www.wma.net/e/policy/17-c_e.html [May 30, 2001].

APPENDIX A
Workshop Agenda
June 21-22, 2001

Session 1:
Comparative Advantages and Disadvantages of Longitudinal Community Studies, Panel Studies, and Cohort Studies

Demographic Analysis of Community, Cohort, and Panel Data from Low-Income Countries: Methodological Issues
    Andrew Foster

Responses to Foster paper from various longitudinal approaches:
    Duncan Thomas, Panel studies
    Linda Adair, Cohort studies

    James F. Phillips, Longitudinal community studies

Session 2:
The Value and Contributions of Longitudinal Studies to Science and Policy

Historical Lessons from Cohort and Household Longitudinal Studies
    Barry Popkin

Longitudinal Community Studies: Time to Invest or Time to Cut Back?
    Stephen Tollman

Lessons from Longitudinal Studies in Developed Countries
    Robert J. Willis

Survival of Adult Women in Rural Bangladesh: A 20-year Follow-up Study Based on the Matlab Demographic Surveillance System and the Determinants of Natural Fertility Study
    Jane Menken

    Monica Das Gupta, Discussant

Session 3:
Issues in the Design of Longitudinal Collection

Linked Analyses
    Allan Hill

Demographic Surveillance among the African Urban Poor: Rationale and Challenges
    Pierre Ngom (coauthors: Eliya M. Zulu and Alex C. Ezeh)

Longitudinal Analysis of STDs/HIV/AIDS
    Ties Boerma

    Agnes Quisumbing, Discussant

Session 4:
Capacity Building and Training

Institution Building Through Longitudinal Efforts in Sub-Saharan Africa
    Cheikh Mbacke

Capacity Building in the African Census project
    Tukufu Zuberi

Training Needs and Efforts
   Kenneth Bridbord

Francis Dodoo, Discussant

June 22, 2001

Session 5:
Frontier Issues in Longitudinal Data Collection and Analysis

Integrating Biology into Surveys of Health and Aging: Experiences from the Taiwan Study
   Noreen Goldman and Maxine Weinstein

GIS Applications in Longitudinal Research
   Stephen Matthews

Stan Becker, Discussant

Session 6:
Ethical Issues Specific to Longitudinal Data

Richard Cash, Presenter

Linda Adair, Discussant

Session 7:
Data Access

Longitudinal Data and Data Sharing: An Overview of the Issues
   Chris Bachrach and Jeffery Evans (coauthor)

Wider Accessibility to Longitudinal Datasets: A Framework for Discussing the Issues
   Kobus Herbst

Negotiating for Use of Data/Data Linking
    Tukufu Zuberi

    Martin Vaessen, Discussant

Session 8:
Marshalling Computer Science Innovations for Longitudinal Research

Next-Generation Data Systems for Longitudinal Health and Demographic Studies
    Bruce MacLeod and James Phillips (coauthor)

A Relational Data Model to Manage Longitudinal Population Data
    Sam Clark

APPENDIX B
Workshop Participants
June 21-22, 2001

Linda Adair, Carolina Population Center, University of North Carolina at Chapel Hill
Jacob Adetunji, U.S. Agency for International Development
Fred Arnold, ORC Macro
Chris Bachrach, Demographic and Behavioral Sciences Branch, National Institute of Child Health and Human Development
Stan Becker, School of Hygiene and Public Health, The Johns Hopkins University
Ties Boerma, Carolina Population Center, University of North Carolina at Chapel Hill
Kenneth Bridbord, Division of International Training and Research, Fogarty International Center, National Institutes of Health
Virginia Cain, National Institutes of Health, Office of Behavioral and Social Sciences Research
Richard Cash, Harvard School of Public Health, Department of Population and International Health
Sam Clark, Population Studies Center, University of Pennsylvania
Monica Das Gupta, The World Bank
Francis Dodoo, Vanderbilt University, Department of Sociology
Rafael Flores, International Food Policy Research Institute
Andrew Foster, Department of Economics and Community Health, Brown University

Noreen Goldman, Office of Population Research, Princeton University
Kobus Herbst, Africa Centre for Reproductive Health and Population Studies
Allan Hill, Department of Population and International Health, Harvard School of Public Health
Kevin Kinsella, International Programs Center, U.S. Bureau of the Census
Michael Koenig, Bloomberg School of Public Health, Department of Population and Family Health Sciences, The Johns Hopkins University
Bruce MacLeod, Computer Science Department, University of Southern Maine
Carolyn Makinson, Andrew W. Mellon Foundation
Frederick Makumbi, School of Hygiene and Public Health, The Johns Hopkins University
John Maluccio, International Food Policy Research Institute
Stephen Matthews, Population Research Institute, Pennsylvania State University
Cheikh Mbacke, The Rockefeller Foundation
Jeanne McDermott, Division of International Training and Research, Fogarty International Center, National Institutes of Health
Jane Menken, Institute of Behavioral Sciences, University of Colorado Boulder
Heather Miller, National Institutes of Health, Office of Extramural Research
Pierre Ngom, African Population and Health Research Center
Rachel Nugent, Fogarty International Center, National Institutes of Health
James F. Phillips, The Population Council, New York
Barry Popkin, Carolina Population Center, University of North Carolina at Chapel Hill
Agnes Quisumbing, International Food Policy Research Institute
Richard Suzman, Behavioral and Social Research Program, National Institute on Aging
Duncan Thomas, RAND and Department of Economics, University of California, Los Angeles

Stephen Tollman, School of Public Health, Faculty of Health Sciences, University of the Witwatersrand (Parktown, South Africa)
Martin Vaessen, Macro International
Maxine Weinstein, Center for Population and Health, Georgetown University
Robert J. Willis, Population Studies Center, University of Michigan
Tukufu Zuberi, Department of Sociology, University of Pennsylvania